When
CANCER
STRIKES
a Friend

To Julie:
May you enjoy the
gifts of good health and
friendship now and
always. Fondly,
[signature]

D0150226

When CANCER STRIKES *a Friend*

What to Say, What to Do, and How to Help

Bonnie E. Draeger

Rachel Abram, Editor

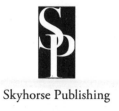

Skyhorse Publishing

All author's profits from the sale of this book will support health care and education initiatives to prevent life-threatening illnesses in at-risk children and families, cancer education, and/or cancer survivor assistance programs. This book is a not-for-profit education initiative of Friends & Cancer (In Marjolein's Memory, Inc.), www.friendsandcancer.org.

Copyright © 2012 by In Marjolein's Memory, Inc.

Artwork on pages 1, 33, 83, and 155 © Sigrid Olsen. Reproduced with permission of the artist.

Cartoons on pages 15, 30, 52, 54, 96, 104, 131, and 147 © Dave Coverly/Distributed by Creators Syndicate, Inc. Reproduced with permission of the artist.

Skyhorse Publishing books may be purchased in bulk at special discounts for sales promotion, corporate gifts, fund-raising, or educational purposes. Special editions can also be created to specifications. For details, contact the Special Sales Department, Skyhorse Publishing, 307 West 36th Street, 11th Floor, New York, NY 10018 or info@skyhorsepublishing.com.

Skyhorse® and Skyhorse Publishing® are registered trademarks of Skyhorse Publishing, Inc.®, a Delaware corporation.

Visit our website at www.skyhorsepublishing.com.

10 9 8 7 6 5 4 3 2 1

Library of Congress Cataloging-in-Publication Data is available on file.

ISBN: 978-1-62087-214-7

Printed in the United States of America

Please note: The information contained in this book is based on personal experience and research and is not, and should not be taken or construed to be, specific legal, medical, or professional advice of any kind or a replacement for professional medical or legal consultation. For legal or medical advice about a specific topic or situation, please consult an attorney or your health care provider. The publisher, author, contributors, and Friends & Cancer (In Marjolein's Memory, Inc.) shall not have any liability or responsibility for any adverse effects or loss caused, or alleged to be caused, directly or indirectly, by any information included in this book.

In Memory of Marjolein Ungerer
and
Rachel Fisher Abram

You each left your imprint on the pages of this book
and upon the lives of all who knew you.

Marjolein, you will be forever remembered
as this book's inspiration.
You dynamically embraced life in the midst of cancer
and passionately advocated on behalf of patients' rights.

Rachel, you will be remembered
as the gifted and insightful editor
who believed in this book and gave it life.
And in the midst of it all,
you were an extraordinary friend.

CONTENTS

INTRODUCTION

You've picked up this book because someone you know has cancer. It may be a close or casual friend, a neighbor or colleague, or even a member of your own extended family. You want to offer your help and support, but you don't know how.

For the past eight years I have listened to the stories and concerns of people just like you. From coast to coast, friends of cancer survivors told me how difficult it was to determine what help was needed and how best to offer it. Like you, they were frustrated by the absence of guidelines and had to figure everything out for themselves. They found numerous books for patients, immediate family members, and primary caregivers, but "Where is the book for friends?" they asked me.

I scoured bookstores, libraries, and Internet sites, but found no book with the guidance friends needed. So I posed the question to five different physicians at New York's Memorial Sloan-Kettering Cancer Center and White Plains Hospital. While the doctors knew of no such book, it was such an important subject that they offered to help me put one together: "Just give us our assignments!"

As news of the project spread, oncologists, physicians, clergy, social workers, and psychologists volunteered to contribute their expertise to the book. A not-for-profit organization, In Marjolein's Memory, Inc.,[1] was formed to oversee the book's research; offer free educational workshops; and assign all profits to health care initiatives for cancer patients, survivors, and children and families at risk of life-threatening illnesses, such as cancer.

I sought the advice and experience of hundreds of survivors and their friends through interviews, questionnaires, and focus groups held nationwide. These participants inspired me, challenged me, and taught me that friends are critically important to patients' well-being. All in all, this continues to be an incredible journey for me, as an author, survivor, and educator.

---

[1] In Marjolein's Memory, Inc., (d/b/a Friends & Cancer) is a registered 501(c)(3) public charity in the state of New York. See www.friendsandcancer.org for more information.

In these pages you will find what cancer experts, survivors, and my own cancer experiences have taught me. This collective wisdom will empower and enable you to lend your very best help and support when cancer strikes a friend.

Using this Book

In the course of researching and preparing this book, I have learned that cancer experiences are as unique and varied as the individuals who struggle with this disease. While there is no single "right way" to respond to friends facing cancer, there are guidelines to help you find countless ways to demonstrate your care and support throughout the cancer journey. The keys are to communicate well, learn about the cancer experience, and assess your friend's needs carefully, so you are then able to offer the best help you can.

This book is designed to provide you with the information and encouragement you need to do just that. It will be a resource you will use again and again, seeking information as you need it. The book is divided into four parts, and you may read them in any order:

Part One, "Finding Your Way as a Friend," presents a basic introduction to the experience of cancer as well as communication tips, guidelines for offering help and setting healthy boundaries, and a list of key cancer facts.

Part Two, "How to Help," defines ten categories of care and support called "gifts of friendship." It provides concrete suggestions for ways to help and support people with cancer through your presence, communication, everyday help, and much more.

Part Three, "When You Want to Know More: The Gift of Knowledge," introduces the modern concept of cancer as a chronic illness and explores the gifts of hope and spiritual care during cancer. It also includes special interest topics: talking to children about cancer, caregivers' needs, cancer in older adults, and more. "Ask the Experts: Cancer Q&A" poses common questions to the experts about biopsies and surgery, chemotherapy and radiation therapy, and complementary integrative approaches.

Part Four, "When Life Draws to a Close," tackles the tough topics of grieving, hospice, and death, as well as sharing the gift of peace, and learning how to become a cancer activist.

This book will move you beyond the initial paralysis and self-doubt so many of us feel when cancer strikes a friend. The following pages are filled with concrete, real-life suggestions that will steer you away from common pitfalls, while providing you with good ideas and sound advice. You will learn how you can improve the life of a friend with cancer through your willingness to step forward and say, "I'm here to help."

PART ONE

FINDING YOUR WAY
AS A FRIEND

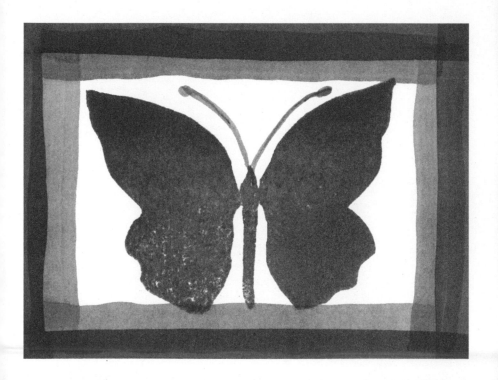

Chapter One

LEARNING TO COMMUNICATE, PREPARING TO HELP

The phone rings and a friend shares the awful news: "I have cancer." You are stunned—so shocked you can't think. You choke on words, not knowing what to say.

It happened to me just a few months ago. Rachel had helped me with this book for several years, and now we had an offer to publish it. There was still work to do, but Rachel was feeling somewhat under the weather. We postponed our editing session so her doctor could run a few tests. Two days later, she called.

"Hey, Rachel, how are you feeling?" I said.

"Not good," she replied. "In fact—not good at all." She paused. "Bonnie, I have pancreatic cancer."

I was stunned. I wailed, "Oh, Rachel. No!" I regretted my response immediately. Although my outburst was honest and she appreciated the depth of my emotion, my primary focus needed to be on Rachel.

I pulled myself together and quickly thought back over all I had learned while researching this book. In a calmer voice, I went on to say, "I'm so sorry you have to go through this. Now, tell me what the doctor said."

As she began to outline the journey, I vowed we would travel this road together.

"I'm here for you, whatever it takes."

In the world of cancer, one thing is certain: No one should ever face cancer alone. The prevailing question is:

When cancer strikes a friend, how should you respond?

FIND YOUR WAY

The first thing to do is to take a breath and set aside the myths and horror stories we've all heard about cancer. With over thirteen million survivors in the United States alone, cancer is no longer considered a death sentence.[1] Do, however, rein in the impulse to announce, "You'll be fine" (even though this is your sincerest hope). Such words can feel dismissive as they belittle what people with cancer are facing and feeling.

Respond to your friend with honesty and sincerity. But remember, friends with cancer do not want pity or long-faced renderings of "I'm *so-o-o-o-o* sorry you're sick." Instead, one of the best responses is to say, "I'm sorry you have to go through this," adding one of the following:

a) "I can't imagine what you must be feeling right now."
b) "You must be overwhelmed."
c) "Tell me what the doctor said."
d) "What's next?"

Sometimes you'll learn of the diagnosis secondhand, and this calls for a different response. Here you can successfully communicate by simply sending the message, "We're thinking of you," as soon as possible. Use voice mail, e-mail, greeting card, or text message and *be certain to add,* "No need to reply to this message. We just wanted you to know you are in our thoughts (and prayers)."

---

[1] The American Cancer Society estimated the number of people in the United States living with a history of cancer totaled 13.7 million in January 2012. It further estimated survivors will number 18 million by 2022. American Cancer Society, *Cancer Treatment & Survivorship Facts & Figures 2012–2013*, Atlanta, 2012.

Later you may want to follow-up with another note, card, or small gift. Very close friends will want to speak to their friend immediately, and may ask if a *short* visit would be appreciated, and when. When you do speak to your friend, sooner or later, by phone or in person, use these tips[2] to guide your conversations:

1. Use language that emphasizes the strength of your relationship and your ongoing support. Communicate your confidence that both of you can handle whatever the future holds. Indicate in your own words, "I'll be here for you."

2. Find ways to communicate to your friend that, "You are still you, cancer or no cancer." Cancer is not *who* your friend is, but *what* your friend is experiencing. Continue to talk about your shared interests, current events, and family news, as well as the latest test findings or chemo treatments. Though your friend's current experiences are colored by cancer, no one wants to be defined by his or her disease.

3. Replace the standard greeting, "How are you?" with "How are you doing today?" The former puts patients on the spot, calling for information that they may not want to share or repeat in casual conversation. The latter enables patients to determine exactly how much information they want, or need, to share with a particular friend on that day.

4. When you simply cannot find the words you need or want, it's perfectly all right to tell your friend, "I don't know what to say" or "I wish I knew what to say."

A word of communication wisdom: During the early weeks following a friend's diagnosis, patients and their families are swamped by the need to make important decisions and to process information quickly. They have little time or energy to meet or speak with each and every acquaintance. Do not feel offended or "left out" if your patient-friend can't speak to you personally or

---

[2] This list was compiled by the author in consultation with Janice Ross, MSN, MA, RN, OCN, CBCN, Bloomington, Indiana. Ms. Ross is manager of the Olcott Center for Cancer Education where she counsels people newly diagnosed with cancer, their families, and their friends.

visit with you until several weeks have passed. There will come a time when major decisions have been made, and patients and their families will have more time to spend with others. One person I interviewed summed it up: "When my husband was first diagnosed with cancer, I especially respected people who made clear

The Importance of Language

Within the world of cancer, you will often find language to be emotionally charged. Although it is best to avoid resorting to cancer terminology when introducing or describing someone undergoing cancer, at times it may be necessary to include these references.

To avoid alienating or upsetting someone with cancer, pay attention to exactly how your friend self-describes his or her location on the cancer journey. People experiencing cancer variously describe themselves as *living with cancer, cancer patients, cancer survivors, in remission*, or *NED* (meaning no evidence of disease). Your friends likely will find one term with which they are most comfortable and a host of others that make them uncomfortable or even angry.

To this day I detest it when people use the phrase *in remission* to describe my situation. To me, this suggests cancer is just waiting to reappear. Instead I consider myself to be a *survivor* who is also *living with cancer*. Occasionally I'll use the term NED. Other survivors, however, say "in remission" suits their situation perfectly.

The word *survivor* holds special meaning in the cancer community. Survivorship doesn't mean "free-of-cancer." It means a patient has now begun his or her survivorship journey, wherever it may lead. For a majority of people living or working in the world of cancer, every individual with cancer is considered a survivor from the day of his or her diagnosis.

—*B.*

Communication Tips: What to Say When . . .

1. **Your friend has received or is waiting for test results.**

   a) Ask open-ended questions: "I heard you've had some tests. How did they go?" This enables your friend to respond: "Fine," "So-so," "Great," or "Okay." You've indicated you're aware something is up, and it is your friend's decision how much information to reveal.

   b) If you feel your friend would like to say more, you can ask, "Just so-so?" If the response is short or dismissive, this is probably not a good time. Let your friend know, "Anytime you feel like talking, I'm a good listener."

2. **You are accompanying a friend to the doctor's office.**

   a) "What kinds of questions do you want to ask the doctor today? Would you like me to come in with you and jot down some notes?"

   b) "Would you like to have lunch or coffee after your appointment? We can talk, if you like, about what you/we heard the doctor say."

   c) "It must be hard not to know what happens next."

   d) Close friends may also offer, "Whatever you learn today, we'll see this through together."

3. **A mutual friend asks, "Did you know Mary has cancer?"**

   a) "No, I didn't. I'm sorry to hear that. Did you speak with Mary, or did you hear this from someone else? Are we free to share this information?"

   b) If you feel you are not violating any privacy or friendship boundaries, you might consider contacting (Mary) and saying, "I've heard some unsettling news."

   by Janice Ross, MSN, MA, RN, OCN, CBCN

their support and availability while respecting my family's need for privacy at this time."

LEARN TO LISTEN

While it is important to know what to say and what to avoid in cancer conversation, it is just as important to listen well. When I asked cancer survivors in focus groups and questionnaires to name the most important things to do for a friend with cancer, they consistently replied, "Just listen!"

Listening well during cancer presents special challenges. We may be uncomfortable with what we hear and learn, leading us to steer conversations away from difficult topics or to stop listening altogether. When you take the time to *really listen* to a friend during cancer, you will find it is a gift to both of you.

What Makes a Good Listener?

1. Good listeners focus on what a friend is saying *right now,* rather than thinking about what they would like to say next.
2. Good listeners stay to hear the *hard* things. They avoid shutting down the conversation with "Don't worry . . ."
3. Good listeners make certain they are hearing what is *really* being said. They ask questions or follow up with, "You mean that . . ." or "What I hear you saying is . . ."
4. Good listeners resist the temptation to steer the conversation to their own agendas.
5. Good listeners don't interrupt and don't rush to fill silences. They are patient.

Good listening involves following conversational cues. A survivor, Carol, describes it this way: "After I was diagnosed with ovarian cancer my friend, Suellen, and I would meet and talk for hours about all kinds of things. Sometimes in the middle of a normal conversation about family or current events I'd suddenly switch to my health. You know, cancer has a way of doing that—intruding without invitation or provocation. Without missing a beat, Suellen went right along with the sudden shift in focus. She listened and she followed my lead. Looking back on it now, I realize that in many ways, hers were the greatest gifts I received during my cancer experience."

Suellen was a savvy friend. Her conversations with Carol didn't focus on illness. Instead, she allowed a normal conversation to ebb and flow, with intermittent forays into the world of cancer. This enabled Carol to process her diagnosis and talk about it at her own pace.

EVALUATE THE SITUATION

Once you are aware of your friend's cancer diagnosis, it's time to explore how you may be able to help. To do this, you'll need to evaluate the situation on two levels: why do you want to help, and what help is truly needed?

Cancer—A Private Affair

In some age groups and cultures, cancer information is not shared openly. For some individuals, cancer remains a strictly private affair. I learned this from Pamela, an elegant, seventy-year-old African American woman who struggled with lung cancer for years.

One day, when Pamela was experiencing a feisty cancer recurrence, I ran into her adult daughter and asked, "How is your mother doing? I'd like to help."

She frowned slightly and took a step back from me. "Mother doesn't air her dirty laundry in public," she said.

"Oh, I see," I mumbled, somewhat taken aback.

Around the same time, a mutual friend, Karen, asked if Pamela would appreciate flowers. "Oh, no, no!" her daughter replied, shaking her head. Pamela didn't want us to acknowledge her disease or provide any help.

Karen and I were stymied. How could we respect Pamela's privacy and still convey our concern and affection? We talked it over and decided to send her cards that said,

"I'm thinking of you" instead of "Get well soon." Later Karen told me, "I noticed each Sunday after I sent a card, Pamela would seek me out following church to inquire about my family—never once mentioning her health." We took this as a thank you, and we stayed in touch with Pamela until her death many years later.

—*B.*

When we learn that someone has cancer, we often feel compelled to help—to do something, and do it now! Psychologist Martha Pierce says we feel this way because deep down we're frightened. Instead of confronting mortality, our friends' or our own, we attempt to scare it away by springing into action.[3]

As a pastor, I found myself in this very situation ten years ago. One Sunday in April, as I shook hands following the worship service, a tall and strikingly beautiful woman in her thirties stood before me. Marilyn and her young daughter, Heidi, always participated enthusiastically in the children's sermon time.

"I'd like to make an appointment to come and see you as soon as possible," she said.

At nine o'clock the next morning, Marilyn walked into my small office and sat down on the loveseat across from me. I didn't know her well, but she impressed me as a strong woman, and I knew she was a popular realtor. This morning her face was somber. I asked, "Is there something you'd like to talk about?"

She lowered her head. "If I tell you, I'll cry," she answered.

I pointed to the two boxes of tissues on my desk. "There's one for you and one for me," I said.

Marilyn began to speak. "I had breast cancer several years ago. Things were fine and we had a baby. Heidi's now two and a half and the cancer is back."

---

[3] Martha Pierce, PhD, a psychologist in private practice in New York, in discussions with the author, New York City, 2005–2006.

As tears trickled down her cheeks, I fought the urge to jump in and try to make it alright.

My mind raced. This lovely woman was sick. What help did she need—childcare for her daughter? Rides to and from treatment? Meal deliveries? Before I went any further, my counseling training kicked in, and I paused to consider a few key questions:

1.   What help was Marilyn actually seeking, if any?
2.   Did I want to help because it was expected of me as her pastor or as a new friend?
3.   Am I someone who always feels the need to step in and help?

In other words, was I seeking to fulfill her needs or mine if I jumped in right now? Marilyn set me straight before I uttered a word.

She smiled and said, "I want to have Heidi baptized, and I would like you to be her godmother."

I was delighted, and at the same time, chagrined. How could I have been so far off?

"Of course," I replied.

I had fallen into a common trap and made an assumption that Marilyn was unable to handle her own illness and needed my help.

Nothing could have been further from the truth. At this point, Marilyn didn't want or need special help. She was dealing with her illness by getting on with her life. She was planning birthday parties and a baptism—celebrating life in the face of recurring cancer.

The day would come, as Marilyn's illness progressed, when she would need and request a great deal of help. But not today.

Every patient deals with cancer in his or her own unique way. As you assess what help and support your friend might need, keep in mind that people with cancer have families and jobs, birthdays and anniversaries—as well as cancer. It is always wise to take a moment to carefully size up the situation before moving ahead.

One way to size up the situation is to ask the following questions:

- What help has my friend requested, if any?
- Will he ask for the help he needs, or will I need to inquire—carefully—about what help he would appreciate when the need for help becomes apparent?
- Am I ready to honor and accept my friend's answers of either "yes" or "no" when I offer help?
- Finally, does my friend already have a large *help network* of family, friends, faith, or professional communities? Do I need to contact a "gatekeeper," that is, someone my friend has chosen to communicate his or her needs to others, or to accept and record offers of help?

As one friend said, "Look to see what people already have available to them. Take the 'lay of the Land of Help' and then—where a gap is visible—offer what you can provide." Once you are reasonably certain your friend will need assistance, take a fresh look at the ways you can and would like to help. Think about ways you can match your own abilities, talents, and interests with your friend's changing needs.

As I interviewed people across the nation, I heard countless stories of unique matches between patients' needs and their friends' abilities to help—from cleaning gutters and wrapping holiday gifts to driving patients four hours (each way) to the best treatment center available. When you devote time or effort on behalf of a friend with cancer, you are sharing a "gift of friendship." As you try to match your friend's needs with what you can provide, avoid common mistakes by considering your strengths, interests, and limitations.

- What things do I naturally enjoy doing with or for others?
- What service can I uniquely provide? Can any of my professional training or special interests meet a need?
- What limits the extent of my participation—distance, time, family, job?
- Are there certain things I cannot, or would rather not, do?

Now add to the mix the nature of your friendship.

- What things have we always shared or enjoyed doing together?
- Are we close or casual friends?
- Is there any help that would be unwelcome or considered "over the top?"

Ground Rules for Offering Help

When I underwent treatment for cancer, I fielded countless phone calls from well-meaning friends who had no idea how to successfully communicate their desire to help. The people I most appreciated—and whose help I most often accepted—followed four ground rules. They were specific, certain, considerate, and willing to accept *no* for an answer.

Be Specific: "'Call me with whatever you need' is really not a helpful offer," said survivors. It places additional responsibility on families and patients who are already overwhelmed. Instead, be specific in your offers of help. For example, call and say, "I'm available for transportation on Thursday or Friday this week. Would you like a ride to chemo, or how about carpool help with the kids?"

Be Certain: Offer only the help you are able and willing to provide. Saying "I'll do anything," may result in a request you cannot fulfill, such as providing transportation to treatment when you are scheduled to work.

Be Considerate: The twists and turns of the cancer journey are hard for patients to predict; knowing what they will need is difficult. Give patient-friends time to consider your offers of help while they think about what comes next and what might be needed. Suggest several ways you could help, and say you'll be back in touch in a few days or a week. When you speak again, your friend may accept one of your suggestions or come up with a different request.

Be Prepared to Accept "No" Graciously: If your friend says, "no, thanks," keep the lines of communication open in case the situation changes. Don't take no as an affront. Help may become more acceptable, or even necessary, in the future. *This is not about you*; it is about what is comfortable and appropriate for your friend at this time.

Be prepared to step out of your comfort zone on occasion, risk a mistake, and then try again. In doing so you will grow, as friends, through one of life's most challenging experiences, and you will add new meaning to the special words, Friends for Life.

Chapter Two

UNDERSTANDING THE CANCER EXPERIENCE

MAPPING THE CANCER JOURNEY

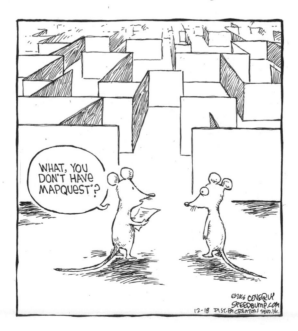

Cancer is uncharted territory for many of us, patients and friends alike. We have little knowledge of what to expect, and we are afraid to ask. In order to provide the help and support patients require, we need a map—a clear and accurate picture of what it means to journey through cancer.

I have asked two nationally recognized cancer practitioners, Alexandra Heerdt, MD, and oncology social worker Rosalind Kleban, to briefly outline the four-phase cancer journey. Dr. Heerdt is a leading breast surgeon at Memorial Sloan-Kettering Cancer Center in New York City. Ms. Kleban is senior clinical supervisor at the Evelyn Lauder Breast Center at Memorial Sloan-Kettering. They will help you understand what it means to experience cancer and will outline the physical and emotional challenges patients often face on the journey.

THE FOUR PHASE JOURNEY

by Alexandra Heerdt, MD, and Rosalind Kleban, MSW

Phase One: Suspicion

While no two cancer journeys are identical, most of them have broad features in common. In general, people respond to a suspicion or a diagnosis of cancer in much the same way they respond to other life stresses. One person will panic and need to see a physician immediately, while another will delay the appointment so he or she can participate in an important event, such as a wedding or a graduation. At some point, however, nearly everyone will experience doubt and fear. In some cases a dose of doubt is important; it allows the patient to go through testing without feeling that a diagnosis of cancer is inevitable. Doubt becomes unhealthy, however, when it prevents someone from proceeding with necessary tests to determine if, in fact, cancer is present. Fear, too, is completely normal and only becomes a problem if it is paralyzing to the patient.

Phase Two: Diagnosis and Testing

When your friend is ready to act on his or her suspicion, the next step will usually include diagnostic testing. Almost certainly there will be blood work and some form of imaging test, such as an MRI, CT scan, or PET scan. Depending on the type of cancer that is suspected, the testing may or may not be invasive. A biopsy may be ordered. It is rare that testing is ever completely without discomfort, and it is likely that more than one test or procedure will be required. This means that test may continue over a period of weeks or even *months*. The testing required for a complete diagnosis and treatment plan may be a journey in itself.

Personality shapes the way we respond emotionally to testing. People who fear invasive procedures will attempt to avoid the tests or will proceed with tremendous anxiety. Other people will go through the motions on autopilot, refusing to acknowledge possible outcomes. This can result in a sense of devastation when cancer is diagnosed.

Some patients can compartmentalize their feelings, and the necessary tests don't significantly affect their other activities. It is unrealistic, however, to think that anyone can entirely ignore the implications of being tested for cancer. Many people find that they are easily distracted and irritable during this time. The uncertainty of the testing period is often harder to accept than the final diagnosis and treatment plan. Some patients say this initial period of waiting is one of the most difficult times in the cancer journey.

The Importance of Distance

While being diagnosed with pancreatic cancer, Rachel looked at her CT scan and spotted the massive tumor on the long tail of the pancreas. "That cancer is a dragon," she declared. The imagery stuck and Rachel's cancer soon became "The Dragon." She emailed friends to share the mantra she had adopted for her journey: "Slay the dragon." I immediately went in search of a dragon-like creature on which to draw a circle with a slash—my own version of "ghost-busting" the disease. I found a multicolored rubber iguana at the zoo and brought it home. Now Rachel's cancer had a face.

Ten years earlier, like Rachel, I had emailed friends to share with them the way in which I was approaching my cancer journey. I wrote,

> "The night before my biopsy, I dreamt a big bear was standing up, peering between the trees on the edge of our property. We called the animal control officer, who proceeded to grill us on the bear's characteristics—size, color, etc. No one was frightened, just determined to get the bear. The next morning I turned to my surgeon as she prepped me for the biopsy and said, 'Dr. Arthur, it doesn't take a graduate degree in psychology to interpret this dream. Go get the Bear.'"

And she did!

Rachel and I each chose a distinctive identity for our cancers because we soon tired of repeating the words "breast cancer" and "pancreatic cancer" over and over. We also chose identities for the cancer to separate it from ourselves. Psychologist Pam Foelsch said, "Instinctively, you did a very wise thing. You created some distance between yourselves and your disease." Assigning cancer a nickname placed *us* in control and helped us to see cancer for what it is: an intrusion, an invasion, an unwanted part of our lives. It enabled us to speak about our disease variously with humor, sarcasm, even anger.

So, when a friend is newly diagnosed with cancer, encourage her to place some distance between herself and the cancer. In this way you will be helping your friend take an early step in claiming control over her cancer experience.

—B.

Phase Three: Treatment

The current approach to treating most cancers often includes a combination of medical disciplines. While some cancers are still treated with one approach, such as surgery, the majority of cancer patients require both surgical and medical management (such as chemotherapy and possibly radiation treatments). The duration of treatment also varies. Some patients require long periods of treatment; others undergo a shorter period of more intense treatment.

Physically, each patient will respond differently. Some patients have a high tolerance for surgical pain. Others will experience significant pain that lingers for some time after the operation. In addition, one patient may feel that chemotherapy and radiation treatments have no effect on his system, while another may have only a few days of feeling "normal" between treatments. The majority of patients have some fatigue during treatment and typically experience other side effects as well.

For most people, the emotional anticipation of impending cancer treatment is as bad as—or even worse than—the treatments themselves. The days and weeks before treatment begins are often filled with intense fear. Your friend's outlook is often informed by the experience of a friend or relative who has undergone cancer treatment. If that outcome or experience was good, optimism prevails; if not, most patients anticipate that treatment will be difficult.

The Courage to Face the Beast

It was a lovely day. Earlier in the week I'd felt well enough to get out a bit. Tonight my husband and I had a table for two reserved at our favorite White Plains restaurant, "Sam's." Looking forward to that evening, however, couldn't change the fact, that I would have chemo in the morning. And although I handled the rest of the three-week cycle reasonably well, this "day before chemo" was always awful. I couldn't focus. Where were my shoes? Where did I set down my watch? What time was I supposed to be ready?

The strange thing was I had no real problems with chemo. I became very ill and seriously dehydrated only once, and that was my own fault. (I neglected to take all the meds prescribed.) This single experience, however, colored my whole approach to treatment; I spent the day before every chemo paralyzed by fear.

However, once the actual treatment day arrived, I perked right up. The infusion center was always bustling with activity. The wait was over and I was ready to face the beast. The oncology staff spurred me on. "You're doing just great; keep it up!" they'd say.

By the end of the day, I returned home proud I'd survived another day of chemo without incident. I would pack the worry away again until next month.

"Chemo really wasn't that bad, after all!" I'd say confidently to my husband.

It's true, cancer is a sly beast. It requires us to summon all we have—and all we are—to fight it, and fight it hard! But I think the times that truly test us are often the quiet times— the times spent anticipating upcoming test results, progress reports, and next-day treatments. We lay in wait. We're preparing to face the beast, one-on-one. And it is during these times of waiting that cancer demands not only patience, but great courage.

—B.

Surgery brings on additional fears. If your friend has never needed major surgery, he or she may have misgivings about the procedure itself and about general anesthesia. Each individual reacts differently to anesthesia, so it is often difficult for a physician to be completely reassuring. Nonetheless, although fears run riot in advance of treatment, the majority of patients do extremely well during their treatment. Unless there are significant complications, the treatment sessions are often reassuring. Patients feel that the cancer is being actively attacked and conquered during this period. Even though there may be significant physical changes during this time, most patients find comfort in being proactive.

Phase Four: Post-Treatment

Almost all cancer patients will be given a schedule of routine post-treatment follow-up visits and/or tests. The timing and details of these requirements will vary according to the type of cancer. As time goes on, some people will be told that they are "cured" of their cancer, while others will be watched indefinitely for any indication of possible recurrence.

For some people, the completion of treatment is a time for celebration. Others, however, find the end of treatment frightening because they are now on their own. And, even though occasionally patients seem to be relatively unaffected by the experience, everyone is affected by having had cancer.

EXPERIENCING POST-TREATMENT: REFLECTIONS ON THE NEW NORMAL

by Bonnie E. Draeger

All cancer survivors hope and pray that the transition from treatment to post-treatment will be their last experience with cancer. This is the time when survivors consider the possibility that a cure has been achieved. But it is also a time full of surprises that make post-treatment one of the most misunderstood and underestimated phases of the cancer journey.

When treatment is complete, cancer survivors are suddenly thrust into a new reality. On the one hand, friends and families are celebrating our successes. "You did it! You survived cancer. Things can finally get back to normal."

The reality is that the "old normal" cannot come back. We have simply moved into another phase of the journey—post-treatment—that has at its heart adapting to a "new normal."

This new normal is a fluid state, changing with the passage of time. It may present us with uncertainties, confidence issues, or the need to adjust to new ways of living. It requires that we let go of the past in order to embrace both the present and future.

For many, the new normal encompasses a monumental change in perspective. The certainties upon which we all base our lives—expectations of good health, long life, career advancement, adequate energy, the possibilities of children or grandchildren—are suddenly called into question: Is the cancer really gone? When will I have the strength to work a full shift? Has my career been negatively affected? Can we or should we have more children? Will I live to see them graduate from high school?

In addition to these uncertainties, for many the start of post-treatment is accompanied by an unwelcome crisis of confidence: Why am I feeling so anxious, so weary and unsettled? I've handled cancer pretty well up until now! In fact, post-treatment is the time when we reflect on the enormity of what has happened to us; we wake up and think, *My God! I had cancer!* These powerful realizations, combined with the abrupt cessation of active cancer-fighting measures, are enough to break down the "can-do" attitude of the most stalwart survivor. For many people, the early post-treatment months are second in stress only to the weeks surrounding their initial diagnosis.

As we transition from patient-survivor to post-treatment survivor, the specter of cancer looms large in the minds of some and stays quietly in the shadows for others. We all want to feel truly cancer-free. Unfortunately, only the lucky few can experience this feeling immediately following treatment. Most of us must wait until our hope is confirmed by years of continued good health. In different ways, we survivors need to accept a new state of being, "living-with-cancer." This may mean "cancer: the memory" or "cancer: the possibility" or both. How are we to navigate all this uncertainty? The best way is to have hope for the future, confidence in our health team, and the ability to adjust and readjust to our fluctuating "new normal."

What constitutes "normal" for each survivor changes from week to week, month to month, and even year to year. The lingering effects and lifelong impacts of facing and surviving cancer influence our perceptions as well as our physical realities. For those completing chemo, the initial new normal may include frustrating memory lapses and a lack of energy. For others, the new normal may mean adjusting emotionally and physically to a radically new body image, to loss of fertility, or new ways of sleeping, moving, or eating. For people whose immune systems have been compromised by months of specialized therapy, such as bone-marrow transplants, "normal" may mean being extremely careful in public, moving away from anyone who coughs or sneezes, and washing hands annoyingly often—for up to a year.

How can friends help? Stick with us; don't back away just yet! If you listen and observe, you can discover clues about what is "too much" exertion or stress for us, and which expectations are unrealistic for the time being. Give us time: time to heal, time to process what has happened to us, and time to prepare to move forward. Living well during post-treatment means embracing and celebrating what we have. It also means coming to grips with what we have lost, replacing sorrow with a deep gratitude for what has been gained—time to live, time to love, and time to enjoy each moment. Celebrate our successes to date, but please recognize we are still on a journey—one that is best traveled in the company of friends.

CHALLENGES ON THE JOURNEY

A Conversation with Pamela Foelsch, PhD

As you accompany your friend through cancer, you will undoubtedly encounter confusing and stressful situations. Becoming aware of these situations and learning appropriate ways to respond to them will prevent additional stress during an already trying time.

Here Pamela Foelsch, PhD, highlights three challenging situations common to cancer. She describes how these situations arise and how to handle them. Dr. Foelsch is a clinical associate professor at the Weill Medical College of Cornell University.

In Sync or Out of Sync?

Situation #1: *Since my friend's diagnosis, our thoughts and feelings are seriously out of sync. Why is this happening and how do I respond appropriately?*

Dr. Foelsch: From the start, there may be a match or mismatch between what you and your patient-friend are thinking and feeling about cancer. A match occurs when the patient's feelings and your own are in sync with each other; you both feel sad, fearful, determined, or optimistic at the same time. A mismatch occurs when you are out of sync with one another's thoughts or feelings. This situation commonly occurs when a patient has already dealt with the initial shock of the diagnosis, but you are hearing the news for the first time. Furthermore, prior experiences, thoughts, and feelings may color what you see in your friend. Perhaps you have lost a friend or relative to cancer, and you are worried you might lose this friend too. The best position is located somewhere in the middle—neither "too matched" where you are both overwhelmed, nor "too mismatched" where you are unable to understand or effectively support your friend. In fact, more often than not, friendship interactions will be a combination of "match" and "mismatch," with the goal of aiming for just the right balance.

This requires several things: to be aware of the situation and to acknowledge and appreciate where each person is *in the present moment*. Be aware of your patient-friend's emotional limits. Don't overwhelm her or complicate her feelings, pushing her out of the delicate balance she has established for herself. It is most important that you take responsibility for your own feelings and reactions to your friend's cancer and *never ask or expect a patient-friend to comfort you!*

Whose Crisis is This?

It was a Saturday night. The phone rang and I heard a familiar voice. "It's Dr. Arthur, and I have your biopsy results," she said.

I gestured to Wayne, my husband, to pick up the office extension. "It's definitely cancer," the surgeon told us, "but it looks like you've caught it early."

We each took a moment to catch our breath and then began asking questions—each of us filling up over three pages of notes. By the time the conversation ended, I was confident we'd caught the cancer in time. Wayne and I hugged each other tightly for a few minutes, and the strength Wayne conveyed through that hug spoke volumes. We would survive this crisis together, as we had survived others before.

I then went downstairs to rework the next morning's children's sermon as Wayne headed to bed—but not to sleep. Retyping the sermon helped me to process what was happening. I finally went to bed around 4:00 AM, exhausted.

After a restless night, Wayne and I got up the next morning and went to church. When the service ended, we began to tell people what we had learned the night before. There were lots of hugs. Though shocked and saddened, all our friends offered helpful words of support and encouragement. All, but one, that is.

Emily and I had worked together on several committees. We knew and admired each other, but were not close friends. That morning, Emily followed me through the church doors and out into the sunlight, her eyes brimming with tears. Before I knew what was happening, this grown woman collapsed into my arms, weeping uncontrollably. I held on to her, trying to offer words of comfort. But in her grief over my diagnosis, she was nearly inconsolable. She finally gathered herself together and apologized softly.

I told her it was okay, but it wasn't. Emily and I were totally out of sync. What was she thinking? I couldn't handle her grief on top of my own. I was holding myself together by a thread.

My astonishment turned to deep disappointment as soon as I got home. Fortunately, it would be a week before I saw

Emily at church again and I trusted that she would have a grip on things by then.

She never fell apart in my presence again, and our friendship endured, even grew. But to this day, I still remember my disappointment in Emily's reaction. I shouldn't have had to take care of anyone but myself on that difficult day.

Changing Boundaries during Cancer

Situation #2: *I have a casual friend with cancer who suddenly wants to become best friends. I don't understand her change in attitude or know how to respond.*

Dr. Foelsch: This situation stems from changing boundaries during cancer. Boundaries are like personal fences that help people differentiate themselves from others. Major life events such as cancer may cause normal boundaries of friendship to change, to become more open. In this situation, your friend has suddenly begun to share more information than had been the norm. She's invited you into her life in a more personal way. This is not unusual, but you shouldn't consider it an invitation to a permanently deeper level of friendship.

How should friends respond to changing boundaries? Stay alert. Things may change quickly. You may find, once the initial shock passes or recovery begins, that your friend will want to return to "business as usual," as if she had never opened up and shared her vulnerability. The intensity of your friendship may suddenly return to its original level. On the other hand, it is possible that, to quote from *Casablanca,* this new relationship could be "the beginning of a beautiful friendship."

Setting Boundaries during Cancer

Situation #3: *We're burned out from helping out. We need guidelines for setting healthy boundaries around the giving and receiving of help during cancer.*

Dr. Foelsch: There is no *should* in being a supportive friend. Some people are willing to be there for others, whether or not their own friendship needs are met. Other friends may feel taken advantage of or depleted as time goes on. As a friend, you need to make decisions regarding your *own* boundaries. Consider the extent to which you are willing and able to be there for your friend. Then decide how much help you are realistically able to provide. Knowing one's own limitations is important. You can only be there in the ways you can be, just as friends with cancer can only accept the help and support they are comfortable receiving.

Neighborhood Burnout

Cindy, a participant in an Illinois focus group, shared this remarkable story about the importance of setting limits.

Our suburban Chicago neighborhood was like a large extended family. We shared carpools and cookouts, birthdays and holidays. It was natural for all of us to come together to help our neighbor, Julie, when she was diagnosed with cancer. During her long illness, we took turns driving her to the doctor, running errands, and providing childcare. We were happy to do it.

When Julie's cancer became terminal, we started making promises. "We'll make certain your family has nutritious meals several times a week," we said.

We prepared a weekly schedule for delivering home-cooked meals to Julie and her family. Then in June, Julie passed away. We continued to bring healthy meals to her husband Jim, and their four children, just as we had promised. Somehow it helped us to keep her memory alive.

After a year and a half, we started to grumble, but guilt prevented us from stopping. We were stuck in a promise.

One night I arrived at Jim's home with dinner in hand. No one was home. After a few minutes, Jim and the kids pulled into the driveway. He jumped out of the car and sheepishly admitted, "We're just getting back from Burger King." Jim was trying to send us a message, but we just didn't hear it.

After this happened a second time, the group met to talk about it. This silliness had gone on long enough! That week, another member of the group went to speak to Jim. "Jim," she said, "I think it's time for us to stop bringing meals. Are you okay with that?" A huge expression of relief spread across Jim's face as he smiled and nodded. Our help had become a burden to him, too, but he didn't know how to say "stop" without hurting our feelings.

We stopped appearing regularly on his doorstep, and Jim began to move on. He even began dating. We were no longer holding him back. The kids moved on too, graduating from elementary, junior high, and senior high school. As Julie's friends, we still kept an eye on the family—but this time from a distance. We accompanied eight-year-old Carl to mother-son events at school and encouraged sixteen-year-old Pete to take his studies seriously. We didn't forget about Julie or her family. We just found new ways to honor our promises to look after them. Our promises now had boundaries— boundaries we could live with.

As a cancer survivor, I firmly agree with Dr. Foelsch's advice. People with cancer don't expect friends and colleagues to upend normal living in order to come to their aid. A little help goes a long way. I strongly suggest that you prevent burnout in two ways: by setting boundaries when you first offer to help and by keeping lines of communication open. For example, when you volunteer to bring meals or provide housekeeping help during chemotherapy, indicate that you'll check back when chemo is completed. At that time, you and your patient-friend can revisit your initial commitment, see what help is still needed, and decide what help you can provide. People with cancer don't expect, or need, unending commitments. Setting realistic boundaries is helpful and healthy both for people living with cancer and the friends who want to help.

As a friend, you will benefit from these strategies in two important ways. They will help reduce stress both for you and your patient-friend. And during the ups and downs of the cancer journey, they will help you maintain and nurture your valued friendship.

The Challenge of Coping:
Attitude versus Authenticity

Most people do cancer in much the same way they do life. We rely on coping mechanisms that have helped us deal with our prior life crises. Some of us use humor or radiate optimism; others employ energizing anger, and still others go through treatment protocols while ignoring cancer as best they can.

Jimmie Holland, MD, says, "When you are in the 'trenches' of cancer treatment, it is best for you to call on the resources you already have."[1]

The mind-body connection is a mysterious and marvelous thing. More and more, science supports the power of the mind, especially when it relates to the body's immune system. No matter how you feel about this issue, there is one thing we all need to remember. No one needs someone insisting that they must maintain a perennially "positive attitude." Positive attitudes may indeed be helpful, but so is occasional anger, fear, or sadness.

"Insisting that [patients] put on a happy face and cope in a way that would be foreign to [them] would actually be an added burden," says Dr. Holland.[2] She calls this the *tyranny of positive thinking*, and this moniker made me stop and think. What right do any of us have to suggest that patient-friends are failures if they can't always be upbeat and positive? Isn't it also important to be honest in dealing with our fears and frustrations?

During cancer, we patients have good days and bad days, and it is important to be authentic in the ways in which we express our feelings, one day to the next. While no one suggests friends should encourage patients to feel sad or defeated, there are some days when it just helps to be able to say out loud, "Cancer sucks," because it does! No amount of optimism or humor can remove that reality.

---

[1] Jimmie C. Holland and Sheldon Lewis, *The Human Side of Cancer: Living with Hope, Coping with Uncertainty* (New York: Quill, 2001), 23.

[2] Ibid., 15.

Every once in a while, patients need a friend who is willing to hear those words, and respond without judgment. Saying, "I just can't imagine . . ." is the truth—and you both know it!

Is there power in positive thinking? Certainly, but it is also empowering for patients to be able to express themselves honestly among friends. And honesty is what friendship is all about.

—B.

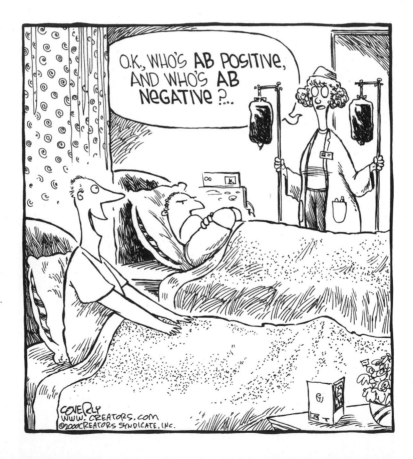

Did You Know? Cancer Facts for Friends

- Cancer is not one, but a group of diseases character-ized by uncontrolled cell division and the spread of abnormal cells. Well over one hundred different types of these diseases have been identified.
- Researchers have identified a number of risk factors for specific cancers and for cancer in general. Common risk factors include: aging; repeated exposure to tobacco, sunlight, or certain chemicals (benzene, asbestos); infectious agents (human papillomavirus, hepatitis B); excessive alcohol use; some hormones; poor nutrition; lack of exercise; obesity; and ioniz-ing radiation. Some people are more sensitive than others to the known risk factors, and some who have cancer have no identifiable risk factors. Having one or more risk factors, however, does not mean you will get cancer.[3]
- Cancer typically occurs in middle-aged and older populations. Over three-quarters (77 percent) of all cancers are diagnosed in patients 55 and older,[4] but cancer can be diagnosed at any age.
- The development of cancer is complex and tends to involve a series of gene mutations that take place over time. These mutations ultimately permit or promote uncontrolled cell division. Some mutations are passed from one generation to the next. However, the American Cancer Society reports that only "about 5% of all cancers are strongly hereditary. . . . Most cancers

---

[3] National Cancer Institute, "What You Need to Know About Cancer" and "Overview," http://www.cancer.gov/cancertopics/wyntk/overview/page3.

[4] American Cancer Society, *Cancer Facts and Figures, 2012* (Atlanta: American Cancer Society), 1.

do not result from inherited genes but from damage to genes occurring during one's lifetime."[5]

- In most cases, cancer causing agents—carcinogens—initiate the mutations. If cancer is to develop, however, this carcinogen must pair with a second agent that promotes cellular transformations, a co-carcinogen. Both must be present for cancer to develop.

- In addition, the body has a natural cancer defense system that includes tumor suppressor genes. The goal of tumor suppressor genes is to repair DNA mistakes. It is important to have these tumor suppressor genes "turned on" to help prevent cancer. When these genes are absent or "turned off," cancer can occur.

by Catherine Sherwood-Laughlin, HSD,
clinical associate professor,
Department of Applied Health Sciences,
Indiana University

---

[5] American Cancer Society, *Cancer Facts and Figures, 2012* (Atlanta: American Cancer Society), 1.

PART TWO

HOW TO HELP: SHARING THE GIFTS OF FRIENDSHIP

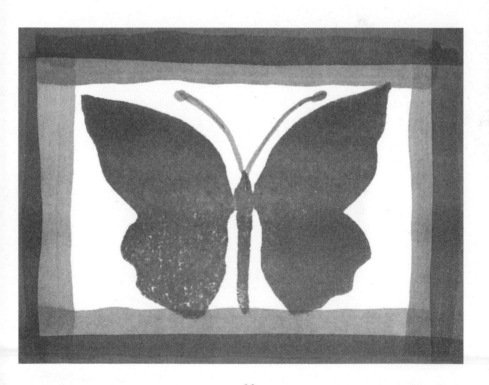

Chapter Three

NORMALCY, PRESENCE, COMMUNICATION, AND DELIGHT

THE GIFTS OF FRIENDSHIP

Whenever a friend devotes time or special effort on behalf of someone with cancer, he or she is providing a unique and powerful gift of friendship. With each phase of cancer survivorship, new opportunities arise to provide needed support and assistance. While there are countless individual gifts of friendship to share during cancer, we will focus on ten broad categories of care and support. The first four categories will be described in this chapter and the others in the chapters to follow. Within each category you will discover a variety of specific ways to creatively meet the needs of patient-survivors and their families.

Ten Gifts of Friendship

Normalcy	Enabling a friend to participate in every-day activities, in spite of limits
Presence	Being there for a friend, emotionally available whether near or far
Communication	Being in touch and staying in touch
Delight	Creating moments of unexpected joy for a friend
Nitty-Gritty	Helping with everyday tasks and chores
Spiritual Care	Meeting your friend's spiritual needs or requests
Knowledge	Researching and sharing requested information
Hope	Sharing a positive state of being, rooted in reality yet transcending it*
Peace	Promoting a sense of wholeness or well-being
Remembrance	Honoring your friendship as a gift beyond limits of space and time

* Vickie Girard first defined hope in this fashion in *There's No Place Like Hope* (Lynnwood, WA: Compendium, Inc., 2004)

GIFTS OF NORMALCY

As every patient knows, cancer is the ultimate out-of-control experience. From day one, cancer disrupts the normal rhythms of life for patients and for their families. During cancer, my life was upended. "My body is falling apart and my whole life is on hold," I complained. I desperately needed elements of normalcy to ground me and to help me regain some semblance of control.

Chapter two introduced the concept of the "new normal" in post-treatment. But what does it mean to experience normalcy *during* treatment? For some, it means being able to enjoy a child's soccer match or a baseball game; for others, it means being able to attend classes or to participate in bridge clubs or book groups. Still others want to continue to work without becoming exhausted or succumbing to dangerous flus and colds.

One of the most heartwarming examples of normalcy is that of Ed, a sixty-nine-year-old softball enthusiast from Cape Cod. When his colon cancer became terminal, senior league teammates invited him to continue playing. "You can do it," they said. "We need you."

In time, Ed became too ill to hit or field balls, so they asked him to coach. For months, Ed's fervor made up for his waning strength. Ed continued to be a "normal," valued participant in the sport he loved, coaching first base until a mere two weeks prior to his death.

How can you encourage this sense of normalcy during cancer? Here are several strategies:

First, behave normally when you're in the presence of people with cancer. "Friends helped me by acting natural," said a survivor. "While realizing that I was coping with cancer, they didn't make that the center of our relationship . . . [Our friendship] did not change and should not change because of illness." This requires us to look beyond illness to see the friends we have always known.

> **Continuing to Contribute**   Arlo was a famous violinist and professor, hospitalized with cancer. His body was failing, but his mind remained keen and strong. Undeterred by his relocation from classroom to hospital, Arlo's students flocked to his bedside for musical coaching. A friend said, "I know this elevated Arlo's spirits, to be considered still a voice to be heard."

> **Out of the Office, but Not Out of the Loop**   Jim was a construction supervisor, well known in his Oregon community as the go-to guy for building information and help. His office was always open to younger staff seeking his experienced counsel. Now Jim was out of the office permanently, confined to his home with terminal cancer. His colleague, Bob, wanted Jim to continue to feel he was still "in the loop," so he called him regularly for advice on upcoming construction issues, even though this same information could easily be obtained at the office.

Next, encourage and implement ways for patients to participate in the routines of daily living *without compromising health or strength*. "We have our good days and bad days just like everyone else," said one survivor. "We're stronger than you think." In social settings, try to meet in healthy venues, e.g., outdoors or away from crowds where germs are least likely to be shared, and refrain from visiting or meeting with patients if you feel ill.

In work settings, encourage flexible schedules that accommodate medical appointments and treatment exhaustion for patients. Find ways to create office environments that protect temporarily weakened immune systems or arrange for temporary telecommuting.

When I was sidelined with cancer, we agreed to hold meetings requiring my attendance at my home—fewer germs, plus bed or bath close at hand when I suffered chemotherapy side effects. The key for friends and coworkers is to remain flexible and be ready to change or adapt plans at the last minute when a patient is having a difficult day.

> **Office Side-Step**   Katy has long been a working mother. Her office desk was always front and center, a hub of workplace activity. After Katy had cancer surgery several years ago, her boss agreed to move her desk temporarily to an out-of-the-way location. She needed fewer contacts with other workers to reduce the possibility of illnesses and infections while undergoing post-surgery chemo treatments. Limiting Katy's contacts in this way enabled her to continue to work and to remain healthy throughout chemotherapy. Later that year when the threat of infection had passed, Katy was able to move her desk back to its former "front and center" location.

> **Substitute Bid**   Ginger loved to play cards but chemo was zapping her strength. Her friends wanted her to continue participating so they decided to bend the rules a bit. Each month an extra player was invited as a "sub." Ginger would play cards and enjoy the company of her friends until she began to tire out. Then, with her blessing, the substitute player took over Ginger's hand while another friend drove her home to rest.

Just Another Wedding Guest

Marilyn received a wedding invitation from her friend Peter. She was eager to attend the celebration in spite of her advancing cancer. By this time, Marilyn was no longer working as a realtor; the cancer had settled deeply into her bones. Some days the pain was unbearable. Family and friends doubted that Marilyn could handle the travel as well as a day of celebrating. However, her desire for normalcy led her to try, and she stoically weathered the three-hour trip and the wedding ceremony.

At the reception, Marilyn's joy eclipsed her pain. As music surrounded her, she danced the night away—totally pain-free. The following week, Marilyn realized that cancer had been the farthest thing from her mind that night. She had felt completely normal—just another wedding guest dancing to the sounds of salsa.

GIFTS OF PRESENCE

"I'll be there for you; you can count on me." This is the bedrock on which all friendships rest. The question is how can you fulfill this promise to be present—*to be there*—during cancer?

Clearly, whenever you provide help in person, you are sharing the gift of your presence. By simply delivering dinner or picking up the kids from school, you are saying, in essence, "I'm here for you."

In this section, we'll focus on intentional acts of presence—those that require a special commitment to provide ongoing emotional availability or physical presence.

How is this done? There are many ways to demonstrate your gift of presence.

1. Make it clear you are emotionally available to patient-friends. This may mean acting as a sounding board, or providing a shoulder to cry on. You can do this in person, by phone, or by electronic means.

Rachel and I worked together for years; we also shared some of cancer's darkest moments. Even though we lived 2,500 miles apart, we made a pact: Whenever either of us would find ourselves at wits' end, we would be in touch and patiently listen to each other, respond with honesty and hope, and *always* look for the humor hidden in the experience.

2. When you are with patients, reassure them that they can try on ideas, process what is happening, or even bemoan their situations *without fear of judgment or critique*. In his book, *On Caring,* Milton Mayerhoff says, "By patiently listening to the distraught man, by being present for him, we give him space to think and feel."[1] This requires additional patience on your part, and occasionally, a willingness to bite your tongue.

    When my friend Evie heard I was considering breast reconstruction following a double mastectomy, she became alarmed and said, "You shouldn't put anything foreign in your body." I explained that this was *my* body, *my* decision, and I expected her to respect my choices. To her credit, Evie never mentioned implants again, and I successfully underwent the procedure *with* her support.

3. Be there in person. Whenever Marilyn had chemotherapy, Karen and I found ways to stop by the chemo center in time to join her for lunch. In the chemotherapy room next door, another patient and her friends often were watching lighthearted movies together. In both instances, the presence of friends underscored the message, "We are in this together."

4. Know the value of touch. Whenever you grasp a hand or offer a hug, you are saying, "I'm here for you." The power of touch speaks volumes. I remember waking after each surgery, reaching up, and grasping the nearest hand. "Just keep holding my hand," I repeated over and over again. Like so many patients, I needed the simple reassurance that I wasn't alone and that someone was there for me.

For some of you, sharing the gift of your presence is intuitive and spontaneous. A sprightly four-year-old taught me this. Our

---

[1] Milton Mayeroff, *On Caring* (New York: HarperPerennial, 1990), 24.

weekly support group was meeting at the church in White Plains. Marilyn walked into the conference room a few minutes late with four-year-old Heidi in tow. There was no baby sitter tonight; Daddy had to work. Heidi had a pink backpack full of crayons and lots of books to keep her busy. Marilyn's cancer was slowly advancing, but she was still working while trying to keep up with an energetic preschooler.

Heidi dropped her backpack and set to work while the adults gathered around the conference table. A lively conversation ensued. The little girl coloring quietly in the corner was all but forgotten. Midway through the discussion, Marilyn blurted out, "I'm worried I won't be able to continue to work much longer. What if I have to go on disability? What if we lose the house? Sometimes I just feel so alone."

We sat in silence grappling for something encouraging to say—but there was nothing. At that very moment Heidi climbed up into the large captain's chair at the head of the table. A few stray bangs fell into her enormous brown eyes. She looked like an angel—and she had heard every word.

Heidi wiggled around in the big chair to face her mother. She smiled broadly as their eyes locked.

"Don't worry, Mommy," she said confidently. "You'll never be alone. You'll always have me." Marilyn took Heidi in her arms and gave her a big hug.

Heidi saw the world as children often do. When she was needed, her presence wasn't an option, it was a given.

Not all of us are as intuitive as Heidi. When you are stumped as to how to demonstrate your gifts of presence, consider these examples from friends and focus group participants.

Calming Presence   While home from college, Kelly offered to drive Bonnie, a recent acquaintance, to her chemo sessions. Kelly was a compassionate listener and a calming presence. While they waited to be called, the new friends chatted about simple, everyday things. When the infusion session finally began, Kelly stayed with Bonnie until the initial anti-nausea drugs took effect. She then politely excused herself to go to work, leaving her new patient-friend calm, centered, and ready to face the day.

The Friendly Tag Team   Cindy was a cancer survivor who lived alone. She wrote, "My dear friends took turns staying with me during the chemo treatments. For the first two days following treatment, one or two of them also stayed at home with me. Then another friend would relieve them." Cindy never had to be alone; there was always someone who loved her close at hand.

Virtual Presence   When Steve's cancer was too advanced for him to join friends for their annual fishing trip, his son-in-law, Stan, took his place. Stan packed a small video camera in with his rod and lures. All through the week, Stan kept an eye out for humorous or thrilling moments to capture on film. Periodically, Steve's old fishing buddies waved at the camera, calling out, "Hello!" or adding colorful comments. When the trip was over, Steve and Stan viewed the footage again and again. Each time, Steve responded to his buddies' remarks as though he were there with them, after all.

Pediatric Presence   Six-year-old Billy was repeatedly hospitalized with low platelet counts during treatment. Billy's first-grade classmates were too young to visit, so they sent hundreds of crayon drawings and messages. As each communication arrived, Billy's parents taped it to a wall in the pediatric unit. Soon there was no more room; the walls were covered from floor to ceiling with hand-drawn pictures, photos, cards, and letters. The colorful presence of these get-well wishes spoke loudly and clearly—"We're with you, Billy!"

Presence from Afar   Thousands of miles separated Regina and Ellen geographically. When Regina was diagnosed with cancer, Ellen sent an email late each night. The following morning Regina would open her computer and find a message from Ellen in her inbox. It said, "Here's your morning HUG! I'm thinking of you. Much love, Ellen."

Listening Presence   When Mary was hospitalized for cancer, she was overwhelmed. The first evening she asked a friend to stay the night at the hospital with her. She was exhausted. Mary needed another person to hear and remember the blizzard of information she was given. Her friend agreed to fill that role. A few days later, Mary left the hospital, more confident now that she knew what was happening and what to expect, thanks to her friend.

Presence often goes well beyond our willingness and availability. In many religions, including Islam, Judaism, and Christianity, lending one's presence during another's illness is not an option, but a sacred responsibility. Anees Shaikh, a leader of the Upper Westchester Muslim Society (Westchester County, New York) points to a beautiful Hadith[2] that says, "A visitor walking to visit a patient will be walking into the mercy of God." It continues, "When the visitor sits with the patient, both will be covered in God's mercy." When we make ourselves emotionally or physically present during another's illness, we are answering the human call to compassion—and for many of us, fulfilling a sacred duty.

The 2:00 AM Friend

I first met Barbara, a cancer survivor, at a wedding. She lives outside Chicago, and at that time, I lived in suburban New York. We hadn't seen each other in over three years when, one night out of the blue, she called me. Barbara had just learned I had cancer.

"I'm here to be your 2:00 AM friend," she said. "You're going to need someone, someday, in the middle of the night. I'm that person. Call or e-mail me anytime."

---

[2] A Hadith is defined as "a narrative record of the sayings or customs of Muhammad and his companions" (*Merriam-Webster's Collegiate Dictionary*, Eleventh Edition, 2008).

Although we barely knew each other, I took Barbara up on her offer. Her emotional availability reassured and comforted me. I knew I would need that 2:00 AM friend one day. In the coming months, whenever steroids kept me up late at night, I found it easy to e-mail Barbara. I asked her how to deal with cancer issues and what to expect next. I used her as a sounding board, and she always responded promptly the next morning.

Her simple offer of presence-from-afar helped me navigate cancer successfully. It also initiated a lifelong friendship.

—B.

GIFTS OF COMMUNICATION

The third gift of friendship is communication. By this I mean getting in touch when learning of a friend's diagnosis and staying in touch through treatment and beyond.

Chapter one outlined ways to communicate at the onset of cancer. But once the initial crisis has passed, many friends lose the sense of urgency that propelled their initial contact. When we inadvertently step back, the result is that patients feel isolated and forgotten. As one survivor put it, "all the shouting is over in the first six weeks."

Roberta vowed that wasn't going to happen to her friend, Patty, who was struggling with breast cancer. Although they weren't best friends, the two had served on a committee together for the previous eighteen months and were fond of each other.

On the first of every month, Roberta picked up the phone and called Patty. "I don't want to tire you out," Roberta said. "Just tell me how you are doing today." The two would chat for no more than five minutes when Roberta would announce, "Now, you rest up and take care, my dear. And I'll check back with you again in a month."

And Roberta did just that for well over a year, offering a valued gift of on-going communication and caring.

In seeking to follow Roberta's example you may wonder, "Are there any ground rules I should follow?" The answer is, "yes."

Ground Rules

1. "Do whatever it takes to maintain connection. Stay connected; stay connected; stay connected," says the late author of *Cancer Etiquette,* Rosanne Kalick.[3]

   My friend Peg lives in Indiana, and I'm on the East Coast. We have been friends for decades. Frustrated by the miles separating us during my cancer experience, she vowed to keep in touch regularly. So, every two weeks Peg added my name to her grocery list.

   When she arrived at the store Peg immediately headed toward the greeting card aisle. There she spent ten minutes selecting a humorous card one week and a sentimental one the next. "It was our time together," Peg said. "And it was good for both of us."

   For over a year Peg mailed me a card with a newsy note or newspaper article attached, every second week. We stayed connected in this very personal way, and as many survivors do, I saved her cards along with other correspondence I received during cancer.

2. Engage in conversations and correspondence that reflect the true nature of your relationship. If the two of you were wild and crazy friends before cancer, don't adopt a new, out-of-character contemplative or serious tone. On the other hand, if you always enjoyed heart-to-heart talks, be prepared to shed a few tears together. Kalick says, "If you spoke to your friend about problems with your teenage daughter before the diagnosis, there's no reason to stop now. If you asked advice from your friend about your job, continue that dialogue. The only caveat is that such conversations be based on how the patient feels at that particular moment."[4]

---

[3] Rosanne Kalick, in discussion with the author, White Plains, New York.

[4] Ibid.

3. .Use common sense when sharing stories. Survivors have all heard the comment, "Oh yes, my Aunt Eleanor had your cancer, but she died." In an attempt to connect with patients, we turn to family cancer anecdotes and often realize, too late, that these stories are not helpful. Avoid cancer-treatment war stories and think carefully, even when sharing positive recovery stories. Remember, *every cancer experience is unique!*

4. If you are unsure how to play it, you can always say, "I don't know whether you feel like laughing, crying, or sitting quietly today." Your friend's response will be your cue for humor, tissues, or a quiet chat.

   As I struggled through cancer, my sister, Kathy, wasn't sure how I was feeling one day, so she sent an envelope containing not one, but two greeting cards. The first was inspirational, and the second, humorous. "I didn't know whether you needed a laugh or a hug," she wrote, "so I sent you one of each."

5. Volunteer to organize ongoing communication between patients, extended family, and friends. Offer to manage a phone tree or encourage the patient's family to send out e-mails regularly. They can also post updates on Facebook or the patient website, CaringBridge.org.[5]

6. It is never too late to reconnect during cancer. For months, our builder, Andrew, was unaware I was battling cancer. When he finally learned of my situation, he personally delivered a large bouquet of flowers. Andrew said, "I assumed all the original flowers would be long gone by now," and he was right. In truth, I appreciated these flowers more than all the timely bouquets delivered during my hospitalizations.

---

[5] CaringBridge.org offers free, personal, private websites for people with significant health challenges. Patients post updates on their condition and treatment on their own webpage. Friends receive a password chosen by the patient to enable access to this page. Friends are then invited to post responses and good wishes for the patient. Sites such as CaringBridge enable patients and friends to maintain contact in an efficient and helpful way.

Tips for Visits

Hospital Visits

- Generally, it is best to wait at least twenty-four hours after procedures before making hospital visits, as your friend may still be in pain, drowsy from anesthesia, or anxious about test results.
- Knock gently on the door of the hospital room before entering, whether the door is open or closed. If it's open, ask, "May I come in?" This gives some control to patients who are constantly bombarded with interruptions and for whom life is out of control.
- To prevent stress and fatigue, keep the visit short, no more than about fifteen to twenty minutes.
- Sit, rather than stand. Try to make your visit one of peace, not anxiety.
- Let your friend be in charge of the visit; follow his or her lead. Listen first, question later. Your first visit is generally not the time to discuss major issues—unless your friend wants to do so.
- In a hospital, patients often feel a loss of identity. A gentle kiss on the forehead, a clasp of the hand, even the straightening of a rumpled blanket can bring instant connection and comfort. You might want to help create a collage of photos or bring framed photographs along to the hospital. The photos will help create a private space in an impersonal environment.

Home Visits

Patients are often sent home from the hospital within just a few days. We have to remember that even though they are home, they are still healing, and healing is a slow process.

- Keep the home visits short.

- Call before you come to the house. It's the courteous thing to do and gives your friend the opportunity to say, "I'm a bit tired; can you come tomorrow?"
- Many of us feel more secure visiting our friend at his or her home. We know the surroundings; we are on friendly turf. However, we must remember that we are dealing with someone who has cancer, and patient-friends should not have to entertain us during our visit.
- Be patient with the patient. Fatigue is common. There may be residual pain. In your desire to "be there," don't expect too much from the patient.
- We need to respond to the cues we see or hear. Most important, create a climate where your friend can say, "Thanks for the visit; time for my nap."

by Rosanne Kalick, MA, MLS

GIFTS OF DELIGHT

Delight is the last thing on a patient's mind during cancer. Here is an opportunity for you to surprise your patient-friend with some unexpected laughter and joy. Author Norman Cousins reminds us in his book *Anatomy of an Illness*, "There is always a margin within which life can be lived with meaning and even with a certain measure of joy, despite illness."[6]

Hospital Heroes

Linda spent day after day at her young son's hospital bedside in Jacksonville, Florida. Six-year-old Matt was being treated for Wilm's Tumor, a childhood kidney cancer.

---

[6] Norman Cousins, *Anatomy of An Illness* (New York: W.W. Norton & Company, Inc., 1979), 167.

One day Linda arrived a bit late, surprised to find her son's hospital corridor filled with paper airplanes, some on the floor and others in flight. In the midst of the chaos sat little Matt in his striped hospital PJ's, holding tightly onto his IV pole.

For days this little aviator had painstakingly folded each and every airplane. His efforts had not gone unnoticed. Now, one by one, his creations became airborne, flying up and down the white tiled corridor—launched and retrieved by half a dozen doctors dressed in scrubs. It was impossible to tell who was more delighted—Matt or the docs!

—*B*.

Creating moments of joy can be as simple as scouring local bakeries for the perfect chocoholic's delight, or as ambitious as making dreams come true. I remember my final day of chemotherapy not for its unpleasantness, but for its delight and humor. A friend, Kelly, schlepped a huge bakery box into the treatment center that day. As she set it down and dramatically opened the lid, everyone stared, wide-eyed. Instead of our usual fare of crackers and clear liquids, we were face-to-face with the biggest chocolate dessert I'd ever seen. As she served patients and staff, Kelly threw in a bit of humor. "The baker calls it Chocolate Decadence," she said, "but Bonnie and I call it Death by Chocolate!"

Las Vegas Dream

Nancy lived in Columbus, Indiana. She had a circle of friends whose actions exemplify those of friends across the country— friends who are quietly making dreams come true.

Nancy told me that one day she decided to join her circle of friends for lunch, even though at the time, her cancer was feisty. The conversation turned to what each woman would do if time and money were no object. Nancy shared her dream of hearing her favorite recording artist live in concert.

When she briefly left the table, Nancy's friends turned to one another and vowed to make her dream come true.

Enlisting help from others in their community, these friends quietly raised sufficient funds to send Nancy and her husband to Las Vegas to see her favorite singer in concert. Then they went a step further. Working with the hotel, they arranged for Nancy to meet the performer just before the show.

The evening of the concert arrived, and Nancy and her husband met the artist in her private quarters. After some time together, this compassionate artist was so moved that she dedicated the evening's performance, in part, to Nancy.

"This experience was the most wonderful gift I received during cancer," Nancy said. "I still can't believe it happened."

—B.

Delight takes many forms. Here are a few suggestions for using delight to celebrate cancer milestones, break up treatment tedium, and brighten patients' days.

1. Find ways to celebrate treatment milestones. Following a friend's surgery (or a particularly difficult time) send a mug, plaque, or teddy bear that says, "You're my hero." Schedule a 50 percent party when your friend is halfway through treatment, and/or plan something special when treatment ends. Whether it's a special dessert, a "girls' night out," or the promise of a romantic dinner, the end of treatment is especially worthy of note.

2. Don't be afraid of humor. There are a times during cancer when humor can be a godsend. Treatment is one of these times. I remember two delightful older ladies, Cynthia and Alice, who in spite of their advancing ages, maintained a certain mischievous streak. Somehow they learned I would be away at a doctor's appointment one day in August, just prior to starting chemotherapy.

In the early afternoon, these two seventy-five-year-olds canvassed my neighborhood until they were certain I had left, and then pulled into my driveway. While Alice remained in the aging Oldsmobile with the motor running, Cynthia hopped out and began to line the front walk with half a dozen large pink flamingos. Before the neighbors could report any "suspicious behavior," Cynthia finished up and ran back to the car. A moment later the two roared off, gravel flying.

When I arrived home late in the afternoon, I did a double-take and burst out laughing. Who could have known this was just the boost I needed? Although they were out of place in suburban New York, I decided the birds could stay if only I could find them a slightly less conspicuous location.

The next morning I repositioned the flock directly beneath my dining room window where I would see them every morning. Those six crazy birds gave me more joy and belly laughs that summer and autumn than I can count. After I completed chemo late that year, I returned the "birds" to their rightful owners, who had finally confessed. I suggested the ladies find them a new home where another cancer patient could receive a daily dose of laughter!

Cancer is serious business, but we don't always have to behave seriously. Psychologist Pamela Foelsch tells us that people with cancer need the humor and the opportunities to laugh that each day brings. Furthermore, Linda MacNeal, CEO of HumorSolutions says, "scientific research has proven that laughing boosts the immune system, relieves stress, stimulates anti-inflammatory agents, releases endorphins to help alleviate pain, and improves sleep."[7]

---

[7] Linda MacNeal, CEO of HumorSolutions, in discussion with the author, Somers, New York, 2004.

There is one caveat, however, says Dr. Foelsch. "You can only help lift spirits when you yourself are feeling able to see the humor in the situation. When you force levity, it only serves to remind patient-friends of their illness, and highlights your own anxiety about their condition."[8]

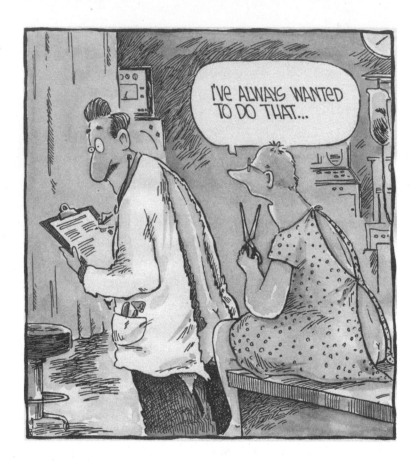

The cancer experience itself is rife with humorous moments, if you and your patient-friend are open to them. One of the funniest moments in my life occurred when I was preparing to undergo reconstructive surgery. Our son was

---

[8] Pamela Foelsch, PhD, in discussion with the author, 2010.

about to be married, and I was midway through the initial phase of breast reconstruction—tissue expansion. In short, there were two little water balloons in my chest that gradually expanded the skin to accommodate future saline implants.

Reconstruction was going well, but I was a little worried. I was in my doctor's office talking with a nurse. "How will I know what size dress to wear to the wedding?" I asked.

"No problem, Bonnie!" she said. "We even do brides. If your dress bodice is too tight, we'll just take a little water out."

"And if it's too loose," I asked, "you'll top off my tanks?" She nodded.

"Well!" I said. "This must be the ultimate in wedding alterations!"

3. Finally, find ways to surround your friend with beauty and make her feel beautiful. Cancer ravages the body and makes it difficult for patients to feel attractive. Whether it's a beautiful silk scarf or free make-up lessons for her, or a classy pair of pajamas for him, finding ways to experience and enjoy beauty during cancer is important.

Movies, Books, Cartoons, and Comedians

Too often, cancer patients receive a boatload of self-help books from well-meaning friends. Instead, author and survivor Betty Aboussie Ellis suggests that friends look for light-hearted movies, books, and cartoons. She also recommends asking patient-survivors, "What movie have you missed that you'd like to see *now that you have the time?*" It may turn out to be a chick-flick, a mystery, or a comedy. Rent or purchase the DVD, then call and offer to drop it off. *If invited*, you can stay and watch it with your friend. Ellis also suggests you inquire about your patient-survivor's favorite comedian, television series, music, or comic strip, and take it from there.*

—*B.*

---

* Betty Aboussie Ellis, author of *Hope, Help and Healing: The Power of Friends and Family in the Fight Against Cancer* (Lenexa, KS), in conversation with the author, 2011.

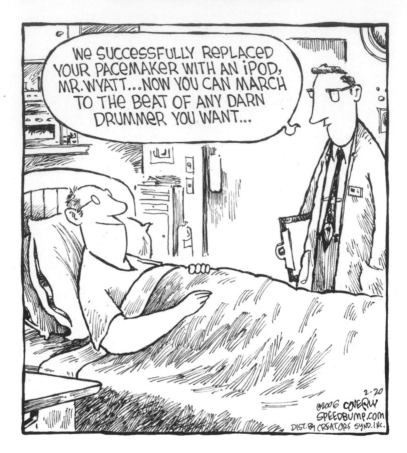

CANCER AND BEAUTY

Artist Sigrid Olsen is a dear friend and a celebrated artist who is well known for her use of vibrant colors and the elements of nature in her paintings, ceramics, and textiles. Many do not know, however, that in the midst of her demanding career, Sigrid Olsen battled breast cancer. Here she shares her inspirational story and thoughts on the role of beauty during cancer.

The Importance of Beauty during Cancer
By Sigrid Olsen

I have come to the conclusion after many years of living that there are very few things of importance in life. But those few things mean everything: love, laughter, human connection, creativity, nature—and beauty, which is found in *all* of these things.

Beauty is at the center of my life. It has provided the purpose for my creative endeavors and the impetus for my career. When I was diagnosed with breast cancer several years ago, I could feel my spirit falling into darkness. There was a place inside me that began to form a dark hard knot of fear. I did everything I could to bring light into that darkness and found that painting and creating beauty had an immense healing effect. So I spent lots of time in my sunlit studio, following my heart. My friends and family helped keep me laughing and happy, and I thank them to this day for that.

But I did have many difficult moments, as I followed the arduous and uncertain path that comes with a breast cancer diagnosis. I will admit that I had concerns for my appearance. It took much searching, but I finally found a surgical team that truly understood my personal need to attain physical health as well as an attractive appearance. After the surgery, every word of praise and delight in my apparent recovery ("You look great!") caused me to feel better and better.

Once I felt well enough after my mastectomy, I started to paint. Creating beauty and sharing it with others has always been my way of feeling beautiful. I literally felt the broken parts inside me rearrange themselves into a pattern of wellness, beauty, and hope. I created a series of work that incorporated uplifting messages with watercolor and print. The work just flowed out of me, and it made me happy to see my inner thoughts and feelings come out onto the paper.

By the end of the summer, I had enough pieces to have a show at my gallery. Friends and customers from all over gathered with me to celebrate my "opening," a celebration of both my recovery and my art. This show of support at the end of my journey was powerful and affirming. As I look back, it is amazing to me now how grateful I am for that time.

SHARING THE GIFTS OF FRIENDSHIP

In this section you will find many meaningful gifts of friendship in the areas of communication, presence, normalcy, and delight (including humor and beauty). They are based on real-life examples shared by survivors, their families, and friends.

Short and Sweet Communication It was the morning after Rosanne's double mastectomy. She was surprised, and not too happy, to see a casual acquaintance enter her hospital room. "I really did not want a visitor," she remembers. "All Lee did was give me a quick kiss and a smile. She had brought a beautiful long stemmed rose, probably from her own garden. Lee placed it on the window ledge and left quietly. The entire visit took less than a minute . . . but the rose sustained me until I went home."

Kids' Communications A family sent Grandpa a tape recorder when they learned of his cancer. The children regularly made and sent creative audiotapes filled with recordings of their music lessons, occasional jokes, and special things they wanted to share with their grandfather. In another instance, young Sierra and Sydney gave their grandmother an iPad so she could stay in touch, in good times and bad. Along with their cousin, Nicky, the three little girls regularly "called" Grandma, and to her delight, she enjoyed not only their voices, but their video presence as well.

Staying Connected Friends made a point of inviting Betty to dinner monthly during her cancer. While she didn't always accept, she wrote, "Invitations to dinner and other social occasions [helped me] to continue to feel connected to ongoing life."

Messy-But-Fun Communications Every third day of chemotherapy, young Andy received a Snoopy greeting card or another cute card. His friends filled the cards with confetti; it was messy, but it was great fun!

Money in Your Pocket Young Charley was hospitalized with cancer in another city. Every time Arlene sent Charley a card or a gift, she added taped-on quarters (dollar bills in today's economy) so Charley and his family could use them in the hospital vending machines whenever someone wanted a snack.

Random Acts of Delight Sam was having dinner at a local restaurant when he spotted Ross's family having dinner at another table. He knew Ross was hospitalized with cancer and that his family was just taking a quick dinner break before heading back. Sam left the restaurant without interrupting them, but managed to stop by the manager's desk on the way out. When Ross's family went to pay their bill, they were told, "It's been taken care of." Sam anonymously had paid the bill.

Childhood Delight In addition to dealing with cancer, Jill was having trouble getting her children's attention, and it was wearing her down. Lexie, just five years old, had overheard Jill discussing the problem with Lexie's mother. She knew just what to do. Lexie went straight to her room and wrapped up three little gifts for Jill: a fairy crown, a wand, and a tinkling bell to call the kids. Lexie delivered her gifts to Jill who laughed with delight and said, "Now, maybe this will do the trick!"

Delightfully "Grand" Eleanor lived in Arizona and was homebound with cancer. It was Christmas and she was looking forward to her grandchildren's visit. As luminarias are a holiday tradition in the Southwest, her neighbors wanted to prepare some for her. They filled dozens of small paper bags with several inches of sand and then set a small votive candle in each.

Just before the children arrived, they lit the candles. Eleanor's walkway was lined with shining luminarias that welcomed the "grands" and delighted Eleanor.

Delicious Delight   Eight-year-old Lauren was hospitalized with cancer. It was summertime, and more than anything, she wanted to have her own lemonade stand. The hospital staff vowed to help her to do just that. Together they created a stand in the hospital corridor just outside Lauren's room. She was delighted whenever nurses and staff would take a break to enjoy her lemonade.

To the Rescue   In rural communities across the county, everyone knows everyone. When word spread that a Montana farmer needed cancer treatment in the midst of the harvest, his neighbors came to the rescue. Twenty combines showed up at his farm, and in less than a day, they cut over 1200 acres, to the owner's relief and joy.

Ongoing Presence   When Evelyn learned Penny had cancer she sent her a brightly colored Asian box. The box had a half-dozen tiny drawers, each containing one small wrapped gift. The instructions were to open one gift each week during treatment and to remember Evelyn was thinking of her. When the box was empty, Penny had a lovely new jewelry box.

Mile High Delight   Harold wanted to help a local family experiencing cancer. He realized the best gift he could give them was airline tickets for a vacation. So he transferred enough of his own frequent flier miles to take care of their tickets. Another donor wanting to help a survivor and his family contributed a vacation time-share as her anonymous gift.

Outrageously Funny Bonnie anticipated she would lose her hair soon due to chemotherapy, so she held an Outrageous Wig Contest. She sent friends and family members emails inviting them to participate. During the next few weeks, folks forwarded Bonnie photos of hilarious wigs that they found on costume internet sites. At the end of the contest,

Bonnie declared a three-foot Beehive wig and a red, blue, and yellow Afro, cowinners.

Humorous "Rescue" To his embarrassment, Stan had trouble getting off the toilet during his illness. His family was sympathetic to his plight but wanted to handle things with a bit of humor. So, one day family members dressed up in helmets, gas masks, rubber gloves, and boots—they flung open the bathroom door and shouted, "We're ready!"

Homemade Humor Chemo left Sarah, a first-grade teacher, completely bald. Sarah's fellow teachers got together and made her a wig out of shredded paper and yarn; they attached it to a hat. Sarah proudly donned her homemade "wig" her first day back at school.

Tacky Trinkets Cancer treatment prevented Sam from joining his colleague, Ed, on a business trip to Asia. Ed went alone, and whenever he had a spare moment, shopped for the tackiest trinkets he could find. At the end of the trip, Ed brought them home to Sam and delivered them with great fanfare. When Sam opened his "gifts," each one cried out "tacky tourist" in its own way. Sam stored his special gifts close at hand in his desk drawer. Whenever cancer became too much, Sam just opened the drawer and received an instant attitude adjustment.

Funny Photos, etc. A friend sent Billy a copy of the hysterically funny *Blue Day Book* by Bradley Trevor Greive, with its photographs of adorable animals in "stressful times." Another friend shared a copy of *Anguished English,* by Richard Lederer. Still another recorded segments of a favorite comedy television series.

Feeling Beautiful A group of friends gave Jeannette a little tree filled with hairpins and hair accessories just as her hair was starting to grow back. Another survivor reported that the nicest gift she received wasn't really a gift at all, but a simple remark, "Dina, you look beautiful."

Beautiful Flowers Mary received an extravagant floral bouquet two days after each of her chemo treatments. These flowers always buoyed her spirits. In time, the anticipation of the bouquets replaced her dread of chemotherapy. (Not all patients are allowed to receive flowers, so check with the hospital, treatment center, or a family member to make certain plants or bouquets are permitted.)

SPECIAL DELIVERIES: GIFTS TO BUY OR SEND

On the following pages you will find a selection of gift ideas to buy or send. You may choose to select a single item, create a themed basket with several items, or shop online for unique gifts. Many of these gifts can be personalized and can be found online. Some are pricey, others are inexpensive. The amount you spend is not important; what is important is to communicate, "I care and I'm thinking of you." Before sending any food items, *ask your friend's family to make you aware of all dietary restrictions he or she may have.*

The Doctor's Notebook The doctor's notebook is one of the most important gifts a friend can provide. Choose an attractive medium sized notebook or journal in which your friend can record important information received during diagnosis and treatment. Suggest he or she take this book to each and every appointment. The patient can jot down questions before doctors' appointments and then the physicians' responses. It is good to add important phone numbers, insurance information, and doctors' contacts to keep them close at hand.

Simple Gifts to Find Online

Teddy Bears
Teddy bears are gifts that delight and comfort cancer patients of all ages. You can shop at Build-A-Bear or order customized bears wearing everything from pajamas to You're-my-Hero superman/superwoman garb from Vermont Teddy Bear (www.vermontteddybear.com).

Gifts and Baskets for Men, Women, and Children

Gifts and specialty baskets are often found in neighborhood floral or card shops. One of the broadest online selections is found at www.healingbaskets.com. This site has humorous, helpful, and inspirational items for anyone with cancer.

Gift Cards

Patients often appreciate pre-paid gift cards for grocery stores, bookstores, pharmacies, restaurants, and online shopping sites. These cards may be purchased at the checkout counter of many retail stores or online.

Skin Care Products

Gentle skin care products are important for people whose skin is compromised by cancer therapies. Such products are available through Lindi Skin (www.lindiskin.com).

Cookies to Send

Cookie bouquets are fun for the whole family. Hand-decorated and/or personalized cookies arranged in a bouquet or container are available from Cookies by Design (www.cookiesbydesign.com).

Themed Baskets

During cancer, I especially appreciated receiving baskets filled with goodies. I found them to be helpful, inspiring, enjoyable, humorous, and/or tasty. These baskets served many purposes, such as the large fruit basket that I emptied and converted to a perfect "bedside basket." When filling a basket, remember to be sensitive to dietary restrictions if you're including food items.

Bedside Basket (mid-sized or large basket, with handle)
When a friend is just home from the hospital, a bedside basket is extremely helpful. The following items may be sent individually or included in the basket:

- a small notebook and pen to record temperatures and medication schedules,
- a thermometer,
- a small box of alcohol wipes,
- travel sized items such as lotion,
- small packages of tissues,

- a small travel alarm to gently remind patients when to take medications,
- a large weekly pill-reminder box with seven to twenty-eight places for medications, and
- a small decorative pillow to hold tightly when coughing and/or to provide comfort for sensitive areas following surgery. (Patients will also want to add their own cell phone, bottled water, and/or favorite paperback book).

Lemon Basket
Lemon is known to ward off nausea. In this basket include items such as lemon hard candies, lemon cookies, bottled lemonade, or lemon herbal tea. You may also add lemon-themed items such as candles, stationery, cloth napkins, or paper goods.

Thank-You Basket—small to medium basket, with handle
This basket can be carried from room to room. It includes a small, pretty journal for recording gifts, food, and volunteer help your friend receives. You can include thank-you notes or stationery, a pen, and stamps. (The patient's address book can be added later.) You may also offer to come back and pick up letters or notes to take to the post office.

Warm-Hugs Basket
This basket of warm clothing may include items such as soft pajamas, hats, or head scarves. Author Rosanne Kalick suggests adding a pair of crazy, colorful socks. Consider including other items, such as a mug filled with packets of herbal teas or specialty cocoas.

Bath Basket (mid-sized to large open basket)
It may be some time before patients can shower following surgery, and a bath basket can perk up sponge baths. Patients with drains can use this basket to store supplies such as alcohol wipes and absorbent pads. You may wish to include small bottles of soothing lotions, a gentle soap, a scented candle, and extra wash cloths.

Literature or Entertainment Basket
This basket includes magazines, paperbacks, a bookstore gift card, a CD by a favorite artist, or a DVD of a favorite movie or TV series.

Chapter Four

EVERYDAY, NITTY-GRITTY HELP

PROVIDING EVERYDAY, NITTY-GRITTY HELP

Friends can make a monumental difference in patients' lives by lending a hand with everyday chores—those simple tasks that consume survivors' precious time and energy. These tasks include everything from making meals and running carpools, to caring for pets, submitting insurance claims, and stringing holiday lights.

This chapter will give you guidelines for choosing and providing routine nitty-gritty help. There are suggestions for bringing tasty and healthy food as well as advice on how to help friends who live alone. But first, to offer the best assistance, you'll need answers to three questions:

1. Who are my friend's gatekeepers?
2. How do I provide help without undermining my friend's independence?
3. What help is appropriate, given the nature of our friendship?

1. Who are my friend's gatekeepers?

In chapter one, I listed ground rules for offering help and suggested you check back later, after patients have considered your initial offer. Calling back once is fine, but I strongly recommend you avoid *repeatedly* phoning patients to ask how, or when, you can help. This becomes taxing for both of you. Instead, ask who will be coordinating help from volunteers.

Many patients convey information, schedule visitors, and coordinate help through the use of "gatekeepers." The primary **Gatekeeper** is a family member or very close friend who has up-to-date information about the patient's condition and schedule. This gatekeeper shares information with friends and family (answering phone calls, initiating a phone tree, sending e-mails, text messaging, or maintaining a patient website such as those found on CaringBridge.com).

The Gatekeeper

In 2002, I was facing three trips to the operating room and months of chemotherapy. I didn't have the energy or time to coordinate all the help I would soon require. I needed a "gatekeeper," someone to jot down my requests for help and then make calls to fill them. So I called my friend, Martha. Although we weren't especially close friends, I respected Martha. She was also someone I could count on to be thoughtful and discreet.

"Would you be willing to act as my gatekeeper?" I asked.

"Sure, I'd be happy to," she responded.

The next time I saw Martha, I handed her my church phone directory. Next to the names of those who had offered help I had written WH—Will Help. This gave Martha a list of potential volunteers.

For several months, she called me each Sunday afternoon to ask what help I needed during the coming week. Once it was a ride to an appointment, another week several meals, and still another, friends to check on me while my husband was out of town. Each week, using the directory, Martha found just the right volunteer to help. As a "third party," Martha enabled volunteers to be frank in saying "yes" or "no" and helped me to save my energy for the more important tasks of healing.

This was a job Martha undertook with style and grace, and was one of the most important roles any friend played during my cancer journey.

—B.

Coordinating volunteers may be part of this gatekeeper's responsibilities or may fall to a second gatekeeper, the **Volunteer Coordinator**. This coordinator records the names and phone numbers of all volunteers and matches them with the patient's requests for help as needed.

The selection of any type of gatekeeper is a highly personal choice made by the patient and his family. If you think you might enjoy one of these roles, try saying, "If you have trouble finding someone to do this, I'll be happy to coordinate volunteers or see that information gets out to friends and family. Just let me know." This places the decision squarely in the patient's hands and will prevent embarrassment if you are not the first choice. In any event, it is important for you to know who is coordinating volunteers and to be in contact with that person. In the absence of any gatekeeper, of course, you will need to contact the patient or her family to offer or schedule your help.[1]

---

[1] Some patients do not have anyone coordinating volunteer help and are trying to do it all themselves. If this is the case, suggest your patient-friend ask a trusted, well-organized friend to take this responsibility off her shoulders.

2. How do I provide help without undermining my friend's independence?

During any serious illness, there is a delicate balance between helping out and usurping a patient's sense of control and independence. During cancer, patients want and need to participate in everyday life—within limits. No cancer patient *wants or needs* all the assistance outlined in this chapter. Surprises are sometimes delightful, but in most instances you should ask before helping out during cancer.

Whether you help once or on a regular basis, take time to consider ways to include patient-survivors, their suggestions, and/or their decisions. For example, when you set out to weed your friend's gardens, ask if she would enjoy supervising or kibitzing while you work. When it is your turn to provide dinner, call to ask, "What tastes good tonight?" In other words, arrange the way in which you provide assistance to allow the individual with cancer to retain some degree of personal control.

Author Rosanne Kalick tells how she accomplished this task. "I'd known my friend Judy for fifty years," says Ms. Kalick. "Now she was recovering at home after cancer surgery, and she called me and said, 'I can only ask this of you. Can you come over and help me clean out my refrigerator?'

That afternoon the two of us worked together. Within an hour, I'd emptied out the contents of the refrigerator, while Judy told me what to keep and what to toss. We put stuff in plastic bags, and Judy labeled everything. What did we accomplish that afternoon? We connected. We reminisced during the entire time. Judy was in control—something very important to people in the cancer zone. I did a lot of listening. We strengthened our friendship, and we ended up with a clean refrigerator."

In my own experience, it was Linda who came to help out during chemotherapy. I had volunteered to make bags of treats for guests attending our son's wedding and wanted to include home-made brownies; Linda offered to help.

One Saturday in October, side-by-side, we baked batch after batch of brownies. Our progress was frequently interrupted by short chemo-induced migraines that required me to stop and rest, with Linda sitting beside me. By the end of the day, we had made and frozen five hundred brownies. More importantly, Linda enabled me to feel that I was an active participant in the wedding preparations, within my physical limits—even though she could easily have completed the task far more efficiently without my "help."

3. What help is appropriate, given the nature of our friendship?

Few people feel comfortable with just anyone cleaning out their refrigerators, cooking in their kitchens, tidying toilets, or sifting through the "bills payable" file. To help you discover what help is appropriate in the context of your friendship, here are two categories of nitty-gritty examples. The first category includes roles appropriate for any friend, coworker, or neighbor. The second category requires a close or special relationship between patients and friends.

Volunteer Roles for Any Friend

Seasonal Help
Grounds Keepers offer to shovel snow or help care for lawns. Others weed or plant patients' gardens.

Seasonal Specialists volunteer to do a change-of-season chore, such as gutter cleaning, putting up holiday lights, or wrapping patients' holiday gifts.

Medical Help
Travel Buddies accompany or drive patients to doctor's appointments, chemotherapy, or radiation treatments, tests, and even surgery.

The Waiting Room Companion offers to keep patients and/or their family members company during long tests and procedures, such as bone scans and surgeries.

Hospital Helpers arrange to spend time at a patient's bedside at home or hospital, giving family members a break to get a quick meal or run errands. Some remain in the hospital overnight, so a patient's spouse can leave to attend to children at home.

Chemo Companions arrange to visit during chemotherapy and remain through part or all of treatment. These friends often bring snacks or lunch, movies, or just news from the neighborhood or workplace.

Pets and Housekeeping

Pet Partners arrange to walk, feed, or care for pets when patients are unable to do so.

Laundry Laborers pick up and return laundry or dry cleaning. They may or may not choose to do the laundry themselves.

Ironing Angels offer a similar service.

Special Times

Vacation Angels donate their sick days or vacation time to colleagues who are ill.

Cancer Activists participate in a cancer-awareness or fundraising event in honor of their patient-friend.

Wish-Come-True-Magicians find ways to uncover a friend's fondest dream and then help make the patient's dream come true.

Food and Family

Errand Runners call before making trips to the post office, dry cleaner, drug store, or card shop to say, "Since I'm on my way to the _____, I'm happy to pick up something for you too."

Grocery Gurus call before going shopping to ask if the patient has a grocery list. They then purchase and deliver listed items. Some grocery gurus also help patients arrange weekly grocery delivery services offered by local markets or supermarkets.

Dinner Deliverers prepare or purchase a meal and deliver it to the patient-survivor and her family.

Volunteer Roles that Require a Special Relationship

Each of the following five roles requires a unique or special relationship between patient and friend. As such, they are not universally appropriate for all friends and colleagues. Before taking on any of them, tactfully inquire if your patient-survivor would like you to assume this responsibility; indicate that if he/she would like your help in another way, that is fine too.

Listener-Recorder-Translators accompany patients to their medical appointments. They listen to doctors and nurses, take notes, and then translate what they see and hear into simple language that patients can understand.

Weekend Warriors stay with patients at home or in the hospital, following surgery or difficult therapies.

The Paperwork Partner assists patient-survivors as they sort through paperwork relating to Medicare or insurance claims, bills, and even household expenses.

Housekeeping Helpers provide nitty-gritty help with housekeeping chores, from cleaning bathrooms and washing floors to changing linens. This help can be offered on a regular or one-time basis. Some friends will help patients find short-term housekeeping help or a professional cleaning service.

Childcare Companions provide special care for patients' children. This care may be offered occasionally or regularly and may include play dates or before-or-after-school childcare. Extended care may be offered on weekends, evenings, or during hospital stays, as family circumstances require.

"Roles" and Little Jane Scott

In their book, *Healing Through Humor*,[2] Charles and Frances Hunter tell the following story about little Jane Scott, titled, "Roles." They write,

> Whenever I'm disappointed with my spot in my life, I stop and think about little Jane Scott. Jane was trying out for a part in a school play. Her mother told me that she'd

---

[2] Charles and Frances Hunter, *Healing Through Humor* (Lake Mary, FL: Creation House Press, 2003), 39.

set her heart on being in it, though she feared she would not be chosen. On the day the parts were awarded, I went with her mother to get Jane after school. Jane rushed up to her mother, eyes shining with pride and excitement. "Guess what, Mom," she shouted. "I've been chosen to clap and cheer."

The Hunters have pointed out a vital truth in cancer, and in life: There are many times when the best thing you can do is to say, "You go, girl," or "Atta-boy." We all need friends who will stand in our corner, ever ready to clap and cheer.

—B.

NITTY-GRITTY HELP WHEN FRIENDS LIVE ALONE

Some patients will require substantially more help than others. This is especially true of people who live alone. I turned to Mary Murphree—a strong, independent, single woman who is also a cancer survivor—to ask for advice. Ms. Murphree is currently a senior advisor at the Center for Women and Work at Rutgers University. When diagnosed with cancer a number of years ago, Murphree was shocked to discover how much help she needed and received from caring friends. Here is her story.

Living Alone with Cancer

by Mary C. Murphree, PhD

Not all cancer patients have families on call. An increasing number of American women and men—across all classes and ethnic groups—are single and living alone. Today, fully 25 percent of all American households are single people over the age of eighteen who live by themselves.[3] Many single men

---

[3] U.S. Census document HH-4

and women will face cancer or other debilitating illnesses in their lives. They range from the older woman living alone to the young person working in a far-away city, from the middle-aged divorcee whose children are away at college to the man or woman whose own parents are too old or infirm to help. When cancer strikes a person living alone, extended family may come to their rescue, but for many single people, there simply are no kin to help them out.

My story is not unique. I was a fifty-seven-year-old single professional woman working and living in New York City. Struck in 1998 with a particularly dangerous ovarian cancer, I faced multiple operations, chemotherapy, and a very long, challenging period leading, hopefully, to full recovery.

What little family I had lived two hundred to two thousand miles away, and I was too sick and incapacitated to even consider traveling from New York to Texas. Furthermore, New York was my home of thirty years, where my job, medical care, and hopes for the future were lodged. Being taken care of by my family was just not a possibility. In a legal and statistical sense, I was essentially "on my own." But, in fact, I was not alone.

Happily, I was blessed with an amazing web of friends, coworkers, and neighbors—friends who became family. In my darkest hours—the emergency room visits, the multiple operations, the chemotherapy, the systemic crashes and step-by-step recovery—through it all, my friends were always there.

Theoretically, there are only three ways for single cancer patients to cope.

(1) They buy their care outright, hiring caretakers left and right, at great cost.

(2) They find assorted health-related social services that provide them a measure of patched care.

(3) Friends and coworkers come to the rescue, divide up the tasks, and act as family.

Most single folks manage with a combination of these three strategies. But it is the love and care of friends in situation after situation that seems to save the day! It is the friends of many singles who become the primary caregivers. For these singles it is safe to say: *It is friends to the rescue.*

In my own case, friends organized themselves into a team and presented themselves "in loco familia," (as my family) to doctors, nurses, and hospital bureaucracy. First, there was Patricia, gatekeeper and volunteer coordinator, who gave assignments to others. She and another friend were links to my blood family, sending them telephone updates and progress reports. Patricia also controlled the number, time, and length of stays of well-meaning friends and acquaintances.

Friends took turns—depending on their work, families, and availability—covering daytime and evening hospital shifts, just to "be" with me. Other friends took detailed notes when doctors came by, fetched x-rays and reports from other hospitals, and tracked down hospital social services. Friends brought fresh nightclothes from home, carried away and did my wash, brought my mail, went to the bank, and brought in special foods to tempt me to eat. Even my new boyfriend (now my long-time sweetheart) took his friendship role seriously, deciding to stick around and take care of me for three more months at home. And so it seems everyone found the thing, big *or* small, that they could do. Will I ever be able to thank them properly? Probably not. Will I ever forget what they did? Never—as long as I live. They are part of my family now and forever.

As for work, my job was my lifeline back to the real world. Friends and colleagues from work did yeoman service during this time. My assistant assumed all my work responsibilities with little additional pay. My boss assured me from Day One that as an employer she would make this work for me, and that my current job was to get well. Later in my recovery, work was arranged so that I could manage from home. The intent was to keep me on the payroll and to keep alive my goals of recovery and returning to work.

Lessons I Learned

by Mary C. Murphree, PhD

Looking back over the years, what advice do I have for those of you with single friends struggling with cancer?

First, **help the single person find social services.** Even well-meaning friends and coworkers can't do it all. Let me repeat: they *can't* do it all! I couldn't bear being 100 percent dependent on the kindness and caring of my friends, but I was too sick and confused to find the services I was entitled to or could afford. It was my friends who worked with the hospital social worker (and each other) to find a nurse's aide to come into my apartment for several hours each day as my surgical wounds healed. And it was my friends who found an affordable RN to supervise in-home shots when I was feeling insecure doing it alone.[4]

Second, **respect the independence of the single man or woman, but take charge if you must.** Single people can be very proud and are by definition independent beings who often need to be in control. To become dependent upon others can be very humiliating to many people, single or not. Asking for help is especially painful. If your friend's family and other support systems are not in evidence, you may have to seize the moment and say, "I am here and I'm ready to take charge *if* you'll let me." Then as the single person gets better and can make his or her own decisions—and resume independence—back off gently. But, *do* back away!

Third, **organize the patient's friends and coworkers to help out as necessary.** Put together a team that will offer a variety of ways to help your friend along the road to recovery. No one friend can do everything, and if they have to, resentment can quickly build up. Many friends make light work; *organize the labors of love!*

---

[4] The National Cancer Institute helps patients and their friends find social services available to help patients once they are home. See: www.cancer.gov/cancertopics/factsheet. Click on "Support, Coping and Resources" and select "Home Care for Cancer Patients" or "How to Find Resources in Your Own Community If You Have Cancer."

When friends come together like this—acting as *family* for singles, younger or older—they provide a lifeline of peace, comfort, and security for the patient. These friends also provide peace of mind for those faraway family members who *do* want to stay in touch but can't do so in person, due to distance, work, or other family obligations.

TEAMWORK

by Bonnie E. Draeger

What I do you cannot do; but what you do, I cannot do. The needs are great, and none of us, including me, ever do great things. But we can do small things, with great love, and together we can do something wonderful.[5]

By now, you have some idea(s) on how you might help out. It's time to decide if you'd prefer to do so individually or as part of a team. Mother Teresa clearly understood the value in a village of help. During cancer, that village requires both organization and cooperation to help prevent turf wars, scheduling snafus, and the duplication of services. The question is: How does one assemble a team that works together efficiently and effectively during cancer?

Organizing and Participating in a Volunteer Team

If your patient-friend is amenable to a team approach, consider hosting an initial meeting for potential volunteers or finding someone else to act as host. If you don't have a ready pool of volunteers, ask the patient's gatekeeper for a list of friends who have offered to help or who are likely to offer their help. Be sure to include the volunteer coordinator if the patient's family has one.

---

[5] Mother Teresa, quoted in *Because You Care*, compiled by Dan Zadra (Lynnwood, WA: Compendium, Inc.), 2005. Reprinted with permission by Compendium, Inc.

At the first meeting, team members should share contact information and talk about the help they are willing and able to provide. This way, if a team member falls ill or has a crisis later on, other potential helpers are already known and on board. At this meeting you will want to:

1. Create a listserv on the Internet. This will enable team members to communicate efficiently with the entire group, check for messages, and respond at their convenience. (If you don't know how to design or use a "listserv," create a group email list and distribute it to all team members.)

2. Take time to consider the needs of your team, both individually and as a group. This may be challenging, but it will enhance the team effort and lessen caregiver burnout, since members are available to support each other. As an example, one member might offer to prepare meals while a second team member volunteers to deliver them.

3. Focus on two essentials: First, the need to provide the best help possible for your friend and his or her family, and second, the need to maintain good relationships among members of the team.

Whether you have organized a team yourself, or have been recruited to participate as a member, here are two tips to make it a successful experience:

Tip #1: Limit unrealistic expectations for yourself and others and throw perfectionism to the winds. While you all want to provide the best care and assistance possible, understand that assistance can be less than perfect and still be successful. The efforts of other team members will not always meet your personal standards of excellence.

Even if you want to, it is unlikely you can bring an exemplary meal every time it is your turn or provide transportation to every radiation treatment. Furthermore, you will find that people with cancer generally see the bigger picture. Little problems and snafus that were once problematic for them no longer seem important. Patients are struggling to survive, and it is of little import in the long run if a dinner arrives a little late or lukewarm.

Tip #2: **Always keep in mind what is most important.** Cancer is stressful for *everyone*. There will always be some disagreements within a team as to what is best. Keep the patient's needs foremost in mind when a disagreement occurs. Try defusing difficult situations with a sense of humor, both towards yourself and others. Move the focus from *efficiency* toward *nurture* and provide help in a way that respects everyone.

When you couple these tips with a large dose of common sense, you will find that teamwork can be a rewarding and effective way to provide a broad spectrum of cancer care without depleting individual helpers' time and energy.[6]

GOOD FRIENDS, GOOD FOOD

Nutrition is not optional. Individuals need to eat, and certainly, the quality and content of the food we eat may be more vital when facing a disease such as cancer.[7]

—*Michael Finkelstein, MD*

To close this chapter I want to address one of the most popular ways to convey care and concern during cancer—bringing food to patients and their families. Unfortunately, we don't necessarily know what foods are appropriate and healthful during cancer. So, I consulted Kristin Kwak—a dietitian-nutrition therapist specializing in nutritional wellness. Ms. Kwak has a special interest in good nutrition during cancer, as she counsels clients and members of her own family who are struggling with this disease. Dr. Michael Finkelstein is the founder and director of SunRaven,

---

[6] "Teamwork" was written in consultation with Julie Willstatter, LCSW (certified psychoanalyst with a private practice in White Plains, NY).

[7] Michael Finkelstein, MD, (SunRaven, Bedford, NY) in discussion with author.

a holistic health center in Bedford, New York. Here are their answers to common questions about nutrition during cancer.

What Can I Bring?

by Kristin Kwak MS, RD, LDN, with
Michael Finkelstein, MD

Since ancient times, the sharing of food has been a universal sign of hospitality and friendship. Food is the medium through which we connect, comfort, and show support. During cancer treatment, nutrition plans are designed to maintain strength and energy, promote healing and recovery, prevent nutritional deficiencies, decrease the risk of infection, and increase tolerance of side effects. Certain side effects may make it difficult for some patients to eat; for this and a number of other reasons, patients may not be able to do everything necessary for good nutrition during this time of crisis. By bringing them sound, nutritious foods, we can encourage healthy eating during cancer.

Below, you will find answers to some of the most frequently asked questions regarding bringing food to people living with cancer.

1. **Will my friend's food preferences and nutritional needs change during cancer?**

   During treatment, there may be times when patients request and tolerate almost all foods, while at other times they have difficulty eating. Food and nutrition needs are likely to vary during cancer treatment, and the desire for food may change as the situation changes. Responding to the situation at hand is the best way to nourish and support friends undergoing treatment.

2. **What guidelines should be followed when bringing food to friends?**

   The rule of thumb is to inquire if your friend has dietary restrictions, special needs, particular food intolerances, or food preferences. Keep in mind that some cancer treatments change the way foods taste, and dishes that were once enjoyable may now be unappealing. Your friend or the primary caregiver can answer the following questions:

1. Has your physician put you on a special diet?
2. Do you have any dietary restrictions?
3. Are there foods that don't agree with you, or just don't taste good?
4. What sounds interesting to you today?
5. Are you open to trying anything new?
6. Would you like me to bring enough for a second meal or for your family?
7. Should I bring food ready to eat or would you prefer to reheat it?

3. How can I choose meals that will provide optimum nutrition?

To help fight your friend's cancer and promote healthy cell growth, focus on bringing foods high in phytochemicals, antioxidants, and bioflavonoids. Translation: structure your meal around plenty of plant-based foods. Purchase and prepare more seasonal, locally grown, colorful whole foods. Incorporate brightly-colored fruits and vegetables like berries, citrus fruits, cantaloupe, kiwi, red grapes, red and green pepper, carrots, dark green lettuce varieties, spinach, sweet potatoes, broccoli, cabbage, onions, and tomatoes. Soy-based foods (like edamame or tofu), legumes, and natural whole grains like brown rice, bulgur, whole wheat couscous, and oatmeal, are good for many patients. Use fresh ingredients and choose organic when possible.

4. In preparing a meal, what should I avoid?

During a course of treatment for cancer or when living with it in remission, the ideal is to feed the body what it needs and to eliminate what is potentially harmful. This is a time for maximum nutrition! Obviously then, junk foods and foods filled with preservatives, hormones, or chemicals (including pesticide exposure) should be avoided. Many processed foods offer far fewer nutrients than whole, fresh products. Diets high in sugar cause cell inflammation and oxidation which results in cell breakdown, aging, and deformation.[8] Read food labels and minimize the use of products that list sugar, high fructose corn syrup, corn syrup, or other sugars among the first three ingredients.

5. **I've heard protein is important for healing and fighting infection. How much is enough?**

Everyone needs protein to fight infection, to repair damaged cells, and to promote healthy tissue growth. Because chemotherapy and other cancer treatments break down cells and tissues, the need for protein increases at least two-fold for people with cancer. It's preferable to include organic, grass-fed beef (lean cuts) and poultry, and to select fresh, cold-water deep-sea fish like wild salmon, halibut, sardines, mackerel, and herring. Sometimes eggs and dairy products are easiest for people to consume; again, choose organic when possible.

6. **Is there room for dessert? I make the BEST brownies!**

Friends with cancer, like other individuals who are ill, are comforted by familiar foods. If you're known for your delicious brownies, wonderful cheesecake, or delectable chocolate chip cookies, consider these as "gifts of love," not nutritious food intended to bolster the body. Try to limit the frequency and amount of these treats and balance them with healthy food or non-food gifts.

7. **What are some alternatives to bringing a meal?**

If you can't cook or just don't have the time, consider the following suggestions:

- Bring a healthy snack basket. Cancer treatment often leaves friends feeling tired and drained, so having small portions of quick pick-me-ups may be just what your friend needs. Individual serving-sized items can be a quick supplement between meals or during those difficult times, a great alternative to eating a full meal. Include fresh or canned fruit

---

[8] *Circulation.* 2009; 120: 1011-20.

in its own syrup (organic is best), almonds, crackers (no hydrogenated fats), low-fat granola, yogurt, whole-grain pretzels, whole-grain cereal, and fluid-replenishing drinks like green tea, lemonade, naturally flavored water, or mineral water.

- Bring your friend a healthy take-out meal. For example, one cancer patient was asked what she would like for dinner; she suggested her friend pick up a roasted chicken and fresh salad greens from a nearby market.
- Dine out. If your friend is feeling up to it and doesn't have any restrictions, it's fine to dine out. Request a table that is far away from the kitchen to avoid cooking smells that may cause nausea or ask to sit outside if it's an option and the weather is good. Avoid fried or greasy foods, and if portion size is a concern, order à-la-carte items. Your friend should make the restaurant aware of any ingredients or foods she cannot tolerate.
- Give your friend a gift certificate to a favorite restaurant. This sends a message of hope and brighter days ahead.
- Create an upbeat dining experience by bringing unscented flowers or candles, balloons, or festive new placemats, napkins, or a tablecloth. Compile a "favorites" music CD to set a positive mood.

8. **What if my friend is nauseated or doesn't have an appetite?**

If nausea or lack of appetite is a problem, encourage ginger tea or peppermint tea or sips of lemonade to ensure adequate hydration. Try making fruit or yogurt-based smoothies to provide calories, protein, and nutrients your friend needs to regain strength, fight infection, and rebuild damaged tissues. Encourage frequent sips of beverages throughout the day to prevent dehydration.[9]

9. **What about herbs and supplements?**

Foods, particularly plant-based foods, contain a wide array of substances that act on the body in many different ways.

---

[9] Nausea or poor nutritional intake that lasts for more than three days should be brought to the attention of your friend's physician.

It is impossible to pack all of the beneficial properties of disease-fighting plant foods into a pill.[10] If your friend is open to it, incorporate foods containing herbs and spices which can help to combat side effects of treatment. *The Cancer-Fighting Kitchen*, by Rebecca Katz, is an excellent resource that can educate and guide you in preparing foods for your friend during this difficult time.[11]

A few final words

If this all sounds daunting, relax. Listen to your friend; let her guide you. Be sensitive and open-minded to her needs and be willing to change or modify plans or recipes if necessary. *Always bring foods in disposable containers* and remember: "Food prepared lovingly will always be lovingly received."[12]

Special Diets and Sample Meals

The body's ability to stay healthy may be compromised during treatment, and certain conditions can arise that warrant a special diet to minimize or improve side effects.

Low residue diet: Residue is the material left in the colon after digestion, including intestinal cells and broken-down food and fiber. Avoid: bran, rice, whole grains; nuts and seeds, popcorn; coconut, dried fruit, fruit skins, apples, berries, citrus fruits, pears, plums, pumpkin, prunes, watermelon; broccoli, cabbage, cauliflower, carrots, peas, rhubarb, squash, tomatoes, and all dairy products.

Sample meal: Chicken breast, boiled parsley potatoes (without skin), green beans, applesauce.

High fiber diet: Fiber is the material in food that doesn't break down during digestion. High fiber diets provide roughage or bulk and must contain at least 25-35 grams of fiber. Five to eight servings of fruits and vegetables and

---

[10] If your friend chooses to take supplements, it's most important that he makes his treatment team aware of the amount and type of all herbs and supplements he is taking.

[11] Rebecca Katz, *The Cancer Fighting Kitchen* (New York: Ten Speed Press, 2009).

[12] Dr. Michael Finkelstein in conversation with Bonnie Draeger, Mt. Kisco, New York.

eight to ten servings of whole grains, plus one to two servings of legumes per day will help to provide enough fiber.

Sample meal: Three-bean chili or bean soup, whole wheat roll, fresh berries with low-fat yogurt.

Low fiber diet: Keep fiber low by choosing foods with less than one gram of fiber per serving (read labels). Rule of thumb is to avoid whole grains, fruits, and vegetables. Acceptable: white bread, white rice and regular pasta, saltine crackers, clear broth, fish, eggs, poultry, meat, and dairy products.

Sample meal: Hot turkey sandwich on a seedless kaiser roll, canned pineapple, fruit-flavored jello.

Liquid diet: A liquid diet may be helpful or necessary during bouts of nausea, vomiting, or diarrhea, or when experiencing mouth sores or difficulty chewing. Ideally, a liquid diet should only be short term and should include products like Ensure, EnsurePlus, or Boost. A major cancer center provides Scandishakes for hospitalized patients. These tasty, high calorie chocolate malts and flavored shakes can also be ordered and prepared for patients recovering at home.

Neutropenic diet: Neutropenia occurs when the white blood cell count becomes very low. It can affect patients who are undergoing bone-marrow transplant or chemotherapy (most often developing seven to ten days after treatment). Neutropenia is a concern because it increases the risk of infection. To decrease risk, be sure to wash your hands before handling foods, and avoid bringing raw or undercooked meat, fish, poultry, and eggs; unpasteurized milk, honey, nuts, fruit and vegetable juices; and all raw vegetables and fruit (except thick-skinned fruits like cantaloupe, oranges, honeydew melon, grapefruit, and bananas which you have carefully washed, peeled, and cut up yourself). Also, stay away from outdated products, moldy foods, and aged cheeses like Brie, sharp cheddar, Camembert, bleu, and feta.

by Kristin Kwak, MS, RD, LDN

PART THREE

WHEN YOU WANT TO KNOW MORE: THE GIFT OF KNOWLEDGE

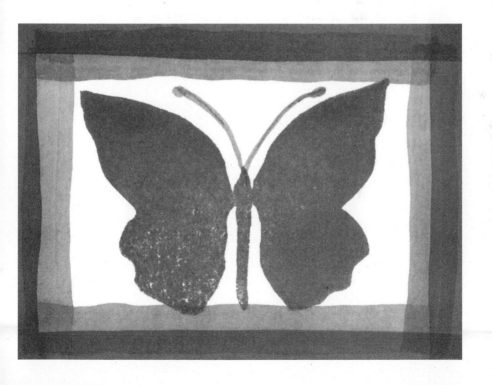

Chapter Five

LIVING WITH CANCER: HOPE AND SPIRITUAL CARE

CANCER AS A CHRONIC DISEASE

People with cancer today are living for longer and longer periods of time. Many of these same people live with cancer as a recurring or chronic disease. Dan Costin, MD, treats patients who are chronically ill with cancer. He is medical director of the Westchester Institute for Treatment of Cancer and Blood Disorders, in White Plains, New York, and a leading oncologist known for his empathic approach toward cancer patients. I have watched him address the fears and concerns of seriously ill patients with wisdom and profound kindness. Here Dr. Costin helps us understand what it means when a friend's cancer returns.

What Friends Should Know
by Dan Costin, MD

"Your cancer has recurred." These are words that no medical oncologist ever finds easy to say and that no cancer patient ever wants to hear. Recurrence signifies a second catastrophic life event. The initial event, the diagnosis of cancer, may have led to treatments with the goal of eradicating the disease so it would never surface again. Stunned by this second event, the survivor may feel incredulous, saddened, betrayed, or defeated.

Why cancer recurs in some patients and not in others is an area of active research. We know that early diagnosis of most cancers, combined with effective multidisciplinary treatment (surgery, chemotherapy, radiation therapy, and others) can dramatically reduce the risk of cancer recurrence. Yet some patients who do *all* the right things and get *all* the best treatments still suffer a recurrence of their illness.

For some patients who have a recurrence, the opportunity for cure may still exist. Careful evaluation of the patient is essential at this time to determine whether aggressive treatments may still be able to eradicate the disease. For other patients, a recurrence may signify that their illness has now become a chronic disease.

With advances in medicine and oncology, it is not unusual to see patients with advanced recurrent cancer live for more than ten years after diagnosis. Some even live twenty years after diagnosis with recurrent or metastatic disease.[1] This potential for longevity and improved quality of life has led to the concept of *cancer as a chronic disease.*

For patients, friends, and family, the idea of cancer as a chronic illness may be difficult to understand. When cancer was first diagnosed, the treatment strategies were generally focused on more aggressive and definitive treatments. Now the goals may change to less aggressive treatments and a greater emphasis on relieving symptoms as well as maximum quality of life.

When cancer recurs, the prognosis can be elusive. We can help by continuing to provide emotional support and comfort to help patient-friends deal with the recurrence. Friends should encourage them to continue with their lives as normally as possible.

---

[1] The *NCI Dictionary of Cancer Terms* describes metastatic as "having to do with metastasis, which is the spread of cancer from the primary site (place where it started) to other places in the body." www.cancer.gov/dictionary. Accessed 10/23/11.

Treatment does not represent a 100-yard dash, but a marathon. Longevity and optimal quality of life—both physical and emotional—are the goals of therapy. Treatment for recurrence may involve additional surgery, chemotherapy, radiation therapy, hormonal therapy, investigational therapy, palliative therapy,[2] or alternative or complementary therapy. Often several of these treatment modalities will be required in the course of treating patients with recurrence.

The hard fact is that when treatment options have finally been exhausted—be it months, years, or decades later—most people who have a recurrence of cancer will eventually succumb to their illness. This is the time when patients can sometimes deal with issues of mortality better than their family and friends. One of the biggest challenges family and friends face is to allow terminally ill patients to face their mortality with honesty and empathy, and not to dissuade them from doing so.

CANCER AND THE GIFT OF HOPE

My second stop after learning I had cancer was a Gilda's Club. Named for comedian Gilda Radner, Gilda's Clubs (now a part of the Cancer Support Community) offer free activity and support groups, classes, counseling, and comfortable surroundings where cancer patients, their families, and friends can gather.[3]

I remember the day I marched up to the front desk of our local Gilda's Club to ask for help. "I've never had cancer before and want to know what to expect," I told the receptionist.

---

[2] Palliation is "relief of symptoms and suffering caused by cancer. . . . Palliation helps a patient feel more comfortable and improves the quality of life, but does not cure the disease," according to the *NCI Dictionary of Cancer Terms*. www.cancer.gov/dictionary. Accessed 10/23/11.

[3] In 2009 Gilda's Clubs Worldwide joined The Wellness Community to become the new Cancer Support Community with over fifty affiliates and one hundred satellite locations, as well as online services. To find the nearest Cancer Support Community, Wellness Community, or Gilda's Club location, search their combined website, www.cancersupportcommunity.org.

After a short orientation session, I was shown to a cozy library. A counselor, Jamie, matter-of-factly asked, "And what are your goals for the coming year?"

Astonished, I replied, "I've just been diagnosed with CANCER; I haven't even thought about it!" I paused and gave it some thought. After a few minutes, I was able to express a new hope. "As a woman of faith, I'd like to go through this experience with as much style and grace as I can muster—and I want to dance at my son's wedding in six months!"

Everyone needs hope, but hope is like clay in the potter's hands. Occasionally it needs to be gently reshaped, as our vision and circumstances change.

"True hope is always based in reality,"[4] says psychologist Elizabeth Clark. "There is no such thing as false hope."[5] This means that a primary task for friends is to find, support, and communicate hope that is rooted in sincerity.

Dr. Clark advises friends to avoid false reassurances, and instead suggests we work to "evaluate the situation realistically and to refocus hope."[6] People with cancer easily recognize hollow reassurances of cure or recovery. When well-meaning friends say, "Oh, you'll be fine!" survivors suppress the impulse to shout, *How do YOU know?*

We also must never lose sight of the importance of hope and the many ways in which hope is fashioned during cancer.[7] Survivor/activist/author Vickie Girard says, "Hope is not a product, but a process. Hope is not contingent on any outcome

---

[4] Used by permission. Elizabeth Clark, *You Have the Right to be Hopeful,* 2nd ed. (Silver Spring, MD: National Coalition for Cancer Survivorship: 1999), 7.

[5] Ibid., 11.

[6] Ibid., 8.

[7] Dr. Elizabeth Clark says, "Health care professionals tend to think in terms of therapeutic hope . . . related to a cure or remission of disease. There is also generalized hope . . . to maintain a high-quality of life despite a cancer diagnosis, and there is particularized hope which is hope for something specific such as being strong enough to walk without crutches at a child's wedding" (Clark, 5). Reprinted by permission of the publisher, the National Coalition for Cancer Survivorship.

. . . Often we must learn that we can be 'well' without being cured."[8]

I saw an example of the dynamic nature of hope when visiting Gary and Carole in Oregon. They live a life infused with hope that is constantly challenged and reshaped by cancer. Gary is an active middle-aged businessman who loves to fish the Northwest's rushing rivers and climb its towering mountains. He lives for the outdoors; he also lives with recurring non-Hodgkins lymphoma.

Gary and his wife accept and understand his cancer as a chronic illness. And while each recurrence brings concerns about life expectancy, Gary's doctors continue to encourage him, saying, "Breakthroughs in cancer research mean that although you will continue to experience recurrences, new treatments will help keep us one step ahead of your cancer."

Occasionally Gary and I talk about his uncertain future, and about life and death. It is clear that Gary and Carole understand that *all is not right* with their world, but they have found ways to be all right *within* that world. They continue to find new hopes. Gary takes more vacation time so they can travel to places they've always wanted to visit—the Mediterranean, Hawaii, and Asia. They are making plans for their future as Carol pursues a new career in landscape design. They live life to the fullest, determined to face that future with confidence and hope—even when cancer recurs, again and again!

Another example is even closer to home. It is that of my mother-in-law, Dorothy Draeger, a retired teacher who lived in rural Watertown, Wisconsin. After being diagnosed with breast cancer in 1971, she participated in studies and in clinical trials at the University of Wisconsin. She lived with recurring metastatic breast cancer for nearly two decades and was an early patient-pioneer in the field of breast cancer treatment. Every three to five years Dorothy's cancer returned—first to her lungs, then to her bones. With each recurrence, Dorothy fought back, taking advantage of the latest treatments available.

---

[8] Vickie Girard, *There's No Place Like Hope*, ed. Dan Zadra. (Lynnwood, WA: Compendium, Inc.) 13, 49. Used with permission by Compendium, Inc.

In time, Dorothy accepted the fact that a cure was not forthcoming, so instead she decided to live a wonderfully full life in spite of her disease. She quilted and gardened, helped out on their farm, was active in her church, and spent lots of time with her grandchildren. She constantly refocused her hope and life on what was important to her.

Cancer was a part of Dorothy's life for over nineteen years, but she never let it rule her life. Her final hope was that her children would accept cancer's inevitable claim on her life, just as she had come to accept it. And it was *her* decision to cease treatment and let cancer run its final course, only after she turned 80—not one day sooner!

Elizabeth Clark tells us, "When a cancer diagnosis is first determined, the individual almost always hopes for a complete cure. If this is not possible, that hope may be transformed into hope for long-term control of the disease, or for extended periods between recurrences. Even when hope for survival is dim, individuals will find other things to hope for—living to see a grandchild born, control of pain, or even a dignified death."[9]

It is the responsibility of each of us to recognize this dynamic and evolving nature of hope and to make it central to the cancer experience—not only for our survivor-friends, but for ourselves as well.

FAITH, SPIRITUALITY, AND CANCER

One way patients and their families face the realities of cancer is to gather strength, hope, and comfort from the teachings of world faith traditions, from Judaism and Christianity, to Islam, Buddhism, and more. As an ordained United Methodist clergywoman, I have seen the interface of faith, spirituality, and cancer firsthand. I have witnessed people who struggled with any concept of God during illness, and I have listened to the many existential questions that arise in the intersection of faith and cancer. Here

---

[9] Clark, *You Have the Right to be Hopeful*, 6. Used by permission of the National Coalition for Cancer Survivorship.

are some guidelines on how to respond when faith and cancer meet head-on:

Making Sense of it All

Many people hold strong religious convictions, and in the face of serious illness, they find that these belief systems offer them significant comfort, encouragement, and inspiration.[10] When faith or spirituality intersect with cancer, however, friends often find themselves perplexed, especially when the patient's beliefs differ from their own.

Life-threatening illnesses often serve as a catalyst for serious spiritual reflection. As certainty unravels, many people want and need to believe that *someone* or *something* is fully in charge, and this cancer is for a purpose. Some living with cancer believe firmly, "This is a part of God's plan for me." Others lash out at God, rejecting long-held beliefs. Still others' theological understanding makes room for ambiguity—living in that puzzling space that exists between limited human experience and complete understanding.

It is often difficult for us to hear spiritual or religious perspectives that we disagree with or do not fully understand. We are all stressed to the max, worried about our patient-friend's survival in this world, much less the next! In spite of this, it is *not* the role of friends to challenge another's dearly held beliefs while he or she is struggling with cancer; as a friend, you need to rein in the temptation to engage in theological debate *unless invited* to do so by your friend. People living with cancer will take the lead in challenging us with profound questions of life or faith when the time is right; take your cues from them. I learned this lesson from Marilyn.

Marilyn came to faith late in life, prodded by the return of her cancer. For nearly three years, she was part of a small group of women that gathered weekly around a worn wooden table in a church conference room. Together we discussed issues of family

---

[10] Others turn to the spirituality of nature, or to community, culture, friends or family, as their primary sources of hope and comfort.

and faith. In the midst of cancer, led by her intellect and her heart, Marilyn repeatedly challenged us emotionally and theologically.

"How can I count on God," she asked, "when my prayers aren't being answered by a remission or a cure? How can God allow this to happen when my daughter Heidi is so young?"

Once, she was so frustrated that she slammed my gift of a New Testament right down on the table, announcing, "These promises are worthless." A few minutes later she said, "I really didn't mean it—the worthless part. Could I please keep the testament and take it home?"

"Of course," I replied.

We understood completely. No one around that table had ready answers that could satisfy a young woman facing terminal cancer. For the most part, we just listened and wondered along with her.

In the midst of her pain, Marilyn's cancer crisis soon became a "window to the Holy" for all of us. As she demanded answers to the unanswerable, we faced life's unfairness together. In the end, it was Marilyn who helped us see life for what it truly is—a fragile, perplexing, and inestimable gift.

Marilyn also led us to deeper understandings of our own faith traditions and helped us move beyond simple acceptance. We discussed the complexities, challenges, and promises of faith. We experienced a Holy Presence supporting us, even as we questioned the reality of that presence. We experienced the peace that faith can impart during pain and suffering. In short, we learned that mature faith includes a willingness to question and explore alongside an openness to experience Divine Encounters that we cannot fully understand.

Blessings and Trials

More often than not, people with cancer experience their disease as a combination of blessings and trials. Survivors say that blessings often include rediscovered relationships, newly understood priorities, and a renewed appreciation for the beauty and fragility of life. People whose lives have been touched by cancer often find new purpose and direction. The question is no longer, "*Why* do I have cancer?" but instead, "*How* has my life taken on new meaning because of my cancer experience?"

Artist Sigrid Olsen said, "I recovered from cancer surgery at home during a particularly lovely summer in seaside Massachusetts. I look back on this time as remarkably beautiful, quiet and introspective . . . where time slowed down and every detail of life was observed with heightened awareness. I sat in the sun on my deck just listening to the birds for hours. I watched the trees sway in the breeze. I drank in the fragrance of flowers that crowded every room, as evidence of the love of friends who cared about me in all corners of the globe. I let my body heal while my mind reveled in the quiet. It is amazing to me now, how grateful I am for that unique time."[11]

Many people of faith also find strength and comfort in a certainty that they are not alone on their journey; they have confidence in the constant presence of the Divine, even in the midst of their pain. Colorado writer and editor Dana Jones talks about her experience of the Divine during her father's cancer journey.

"My father was seriously ill with pancreatic cancer," says Jones. "I tried bargaining with God. I was angry, and I shouted at God . . . 'How can you let this happen?' When I finally came to grips with how sick he was, my prayers stopped. I couldn't find words for the pain. My heart and soul sighed. Not a little, shallow sigh, but a deep, protracted moan.

"Somewhere in that sigh, I felt lifted up. I heard God say, 'You don't need words. I'm with you. I hurt too.' And then I'm sure I heard God sigh so deeply it encompassed my pain. . . . The amazing thing about such sighs is that God hears and accepts them as our deepest prayers. God sighs with us."[12]

---

[11] Sigrid Olsen, in written communication with the author, 2008.

[12] Dana Jones, (Memorial United Methodist Church, White Plains, NY), January 8, 2006.

"WHY?"

Like Dana, we may find ourselves angry at God for allowing our friend to experience such terrible pain and loss. How could this have happened? Why did it happen? Where is the Divine in all this? When we hear patients ask questions like these, they do not want responses such as, "God never gives you more than you can handle."

Hospice chaplain Rev. William Griffith explains. "When people ask, 'Why is this happening to me?' or 'What did I do to deserve this?' they are really wrestling with ultimate issues of identity, meaning, and worth. They are not so much asking for medical documentation or for theological doctrines, as they are sharing their own pain . . . It is natural for friends and family to be frustrated, to feel at a loss because we cannot 'fix it.'"[13]

In trying to understand your friend's situation, you will find there are different viewpoints among world religions regarding adversity, serious illness, and the will of God.[14] As a United Methodist clergywoman and cancer survivor, I am convinced that the *whys* of cancer fall concretely within the realm of biology, not theology. Cancer is a disease—a dis-*ease* in the systems of the body. It is not a friend's role to suggest that anyone acquires cancer by divine will or by familial or personal failure. Cancer is difficult enough to face without friends inadvertently adding guilt to the mix.

---

[13] William Griffith, in discussion with the author, 2006.

[14] Anees Shaikh in written communication and discussion with the author, White Plains, NY, 2007, says,

    (a) "Islam stresses that God has his own wisdom as to why he allows cancer to inflict people."

    (b) "The Islamic perspective on difficulties and adversities in this worldly life is to consider them as a test—a test of faith in God, a test of our gratitude for the blessings in our lives, a test of whether we, as friends of those faced with difficulty, will give comfort and ask God for healing."

Counting Down Chemo

The diagnosis was confirmed, the surgeries were completed, and now I was about to begin sixteen weeks of killer chemotherapy. I knew it would be tough; I needed something to help me keep the end in sight *every day*. So I decided to count down chemo—backwards!

A friend, Lorna, had just given me a book of Psalms that had nice large margins and space between the lines for personal remarks and reflections. I remembered that many psalms were actually laments giving voice to the fears, frustrations, and worries of the ancient Hebrews. Why not my mine? Couldn't I substitute my chemo-complaints for the worries and complaints of the Hebrews?

And so I did. Feeling a bit like Scheherazade, each evening just before bed, I reached for the same book—every night for 112 nights! I began with Psalm 112 and moved steadily toward Psalm 1; I began by taking a pencil and scratching out the psalmist's cause for lament (or joy) and inserting my own instead. One night it was anger at the indignities of chemo's side effects. Another it was the delight in a day filled with energy. Still other nights I wrote of my frustration with a troublesome white blood count, a low red blood count, or both.

After writing my lament in silence, I read the psalm out loud to no one but God and me! And it helped. It helped a lot! I was constantly amazed at how often my deepest thoughts, fears, and small victories mirrored those of the ancient psalmist.

And when I reached Psalm 1, it was a day of pure joy. I had survived another phase of the cancer journey. And I couldn't have done it without the help of my friends, my faith, and the wisdom of some ancient sages.

—*B.*

Gifts of Prayer and Healing

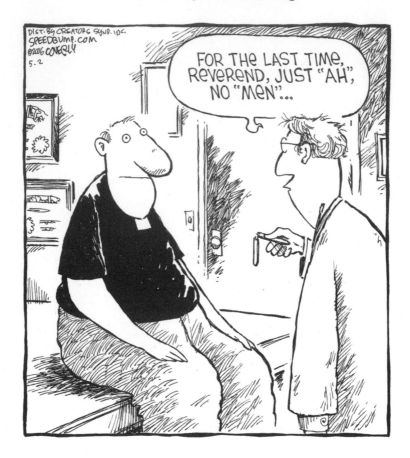

People often remark, "I don't know what to pray for." Our prayers for divine help must be not only for our friend, but also for those entrusted with his or her medical care. A Muslim friend, Anees Shaikh, said, "Pray for the means from God to achieve what is needed for the patient."[15] This means we should include prayers for doctors' insight and accurate diagnoses, for good decisions, and for surgeons with skillful hands. We pray for bodies that will

---

[15] Annes Shaikh in conversation with the author, White Plains, New York, 2007.

respond positively to therapies, surgeries, and treatments—for nurses, hospice workers, and caregivers, that they might *really* listen to our friend and accurately hear what is needed.

If cancer appears terminal, our prayers may turn to the healing of relationships and/or emotional or spiritual rifts. In *The Healing Touch*, Todd Outcalt reminds us that *cure* refers to the absence of disease, while *healing* encompasses physical, mental, emotional, or spiritual wellbeing.[16] Throughout the cancer journey, you can pray for the gift of time for your friend. At the end of the journey you can participate in prayers or meditations seeking peace—peace of body, mind, and spirit for your friend, family members, and yourself.

Often when someone we care about is ill, it is easy to overlook our own physical and emotional needs. Don't forget to pray for your own peace of mind and strength. And finally, pray for the Divine to accompany you every time you enter a hospital, hospice, or home recovery room.

Marilyn's Last Gift

As Marilyn's cancer advanced, she spent more time resting, confined to the living room sofa. Although she required this rest, Marilyn also needed the company and combined energy of her friends. One afternoon, as the shadows of early winter broadened, Marilyn picked up the phone. "Karen," she said, "would you be willing to call together some of our mutual friends and ask them to come over at 6:30?"

"Of course," Karen said, "But what is it you want us to do?"

"I want you all to be part of a prayer circle for me."

Not exactly certain what a "prayer circle" was, but eager to help Marilyn, Karen called about a dozen friends and simply said that Marilyn needed us. We were eager to help.

---

[16] Outcalt, Todd. *The Healing Touch: Experiencing God's Love in the Midst of Our Pain* (Deerfield Beach, FL: Faith Communications, Inc.), 2005.

· At the appointed hour, one by one, we entered Marilyn's quiet and peaceful living room. There Marilyn rested on the worn sofa with her parents standing nearby. She was very weak and had to summon all her strength just to reach out to each friend, receiving hugs and smiles in return.

We all chatted quietly, catching up with one another until Marilyn interrupted us. She spoke softly. "Will you circle around me?" Marilyn asked. "I want you to form a prayer circle."

Somewhat bewildered, we looked at one another and then at Marilyn.

"Here's what we'll do," she said. "Take a few moments and then each of you just say whatever comes to mind, like a prayer."

We all fell silent, and then the meditations of our hearts suddenly took flight. One by one we offered up our deepest prayers for Marilyn's comfort, for her family, and for her peace of mind. Our love for her poured out and we were soon sharing just how much she meant to all of us. It was a powerful time for everyone.

That night we continued to watch Marilyn drift in and out of awareness. Her life was slowly and inevitably drawing to a close, but she knew what she needed—the presence of her friends. Even as Marilyn reached out for our help, we who responded to her request received the greatest gift.

After her death a few weeks later, we all reflected upon that special time together. Even Marilyn's parents, who did not consider themselves religious, remarked that this was one of the most meaningful evenings they had experienced during their daughter's long illness.

—B.

Spiritual Responses: Words

Asking "May I pray for you?" or "May I add you to our congregation's prayer list?" is often deeply appreciated. It is important to *ask*, however, as not everyone is comfortable with public prayer and other spiritual gestures. "I didn't appreciate a woman entering my hospital room and placing crystals under my bed," Mary, a cancer survivor, told me. Never make assumptions about what spiritual practices will be appreciated.

Finally, a hug (with permission and clean hands)—or a smile—can fill a void beautifully when words escape us.

If You are Religious and Your
Friend is Not

"I would like to believe in God, but I just can't," said Carol, after her cancer diagnosis.

Since my own faith had brought great strength and comfort during my illness, I asked her, "How, then, did you get through cancer?"

"I relied on my friends to get me through it," Carol replied.

Not everyone relies on a faith tradition during cancer. Carol's comments reminded me of a basic rule of friendship during cancer: It is our role as friends to support patients fully, even when a patient's beliefs are inconsistent with our own. Regardless of our own religious beliefs, there are many things we can do for our friend to promote hope and spiritual care.

SHARING GIFTS OF HOPE AND
SPIRITUAL CARE

Words of Hope Eleanor was searching for a small gift that was short and inspirational. She looked in countless locations and found it in the hospital bookstore—*There's No Place Like HOPE: A Guide to Beating Cancer in Mind-Sized Bites* by author-survivor Vickie Girard.[17]

---

[17] Vickie Girard, Dan Zadra, ed. There's No Place Like HOPE: A Guide to Beating Cancer in Mind-Sized Bites (Lynnwood, WA: Compendium, Inc., 2004).

Flowering Hope Cheryl's survival was tenuous and she needed a new source of hope. Her friends communicated their confidence in her recovery by planting a flowering apple tree in her yard. "Just you wait and see," they said. "You're going to enjoy apples from that tree one day." And indeed, Cheryl did gain strength as she watched the tree grow and mature, beating all odds!

Light of Hope Michele was in and out of the hospital fighting cancer. Her friends wanted to give her something to "hold on to" literally whenever hope faded. During one stay, friends brought Michele a small flashlight. "Put it on the nightstand," they said, "Then pick it up and turn it on whenever you're having a bad day. This is your light at the end of the tunnel. It's your light of hope."

Inclusive Hope Chris was living with terminal cancer in Bloomington, Indiana. A number of his friends belonged to the local Rotary Club and they hatched a plan. The organization invited Chris to become a new member, in spite of his shortened life expectancy. Their message was clear and strong. Chris was a valued and productive member of the community, cancer or no cancer.

Engaging Hope Jim was a music educator who spent his summers as the director of a Canadian music camp. One summer he booked a terminally ill friend, Eli, to be a guest artist at the festival. Jim knew Eli would likely be unable to perform at the festival, but it was his way of offering Eli hope and encouragement when it was most needed.

Spiritual Presence Lois lived a thousand miles away, but she wanted to remind her sister-in-law of her *presence-from-a-distance*. A talented seamstress and quilter, Lois fashioned a small lap quilt. She took it to church where her friends tied the quilt with small, yarn knots. As each quilter tied her knot, she offered a silent prayer for Bonnie's healing and well-being. They called it a "prayer quilt" and today that quilt remains a beautiful reminder of friends and faith.

Prayer Shawls Hospitals can be chilly and sterile environments. To offset this problem, congregations across the country have formed groups of knitters who create shawls for people with serious illnesses and their family members. They are delivered to people in hospitals and those who are homebound. These shawls enfold their recipients in the love of friends and strangers and often have a special prayer for the recipient attached.

Prayers at the Ancient Wall   The Western Wall in Jerusalem is a location where many believe prayer ascends directly to God. At the Wall, four different friends of Rachel's, who did not know one other, placed prayers of healing, stuffing them into the ancient cracks. Some of the friends lived in Israel, others were visiting. Of course, of greatest importance, they all told Rachel about their visits to the Wall, helping her feel connected to the energy and love expressed in these acts of devotion.

Chapter Six

SPECIAL SITUATIONS

CANCER AND THE CAREGIVER

We are often stymied by a number of special situations that are part of the cancer landscape. I asked Carol Decker, PhD, a research scientist at the Indiana University School of Nursing, to help us recognize the needs of today's cancer caregivers. Dr. Decker's area of expertise is social support, coping, and communication in families facing cancer. Here is her advice on understanding, and helping, today's caregivers:

CAREGIVERS NEED HELP TOO

by Carol Decker, PhD, MSEd, MSW

The people closest to cancer patients—their spouses, partners, parents, adult children, or very close friends—often serve as their caregivers during treatment and recovery. Surprisingly, many caregivers (especially spouses and partners) *experience as much, if not more distress than the cancer survivors themselves*. They are often overwhelmed by a combination of emotional and physical demands, including: the fears and uncertainty that come when a loved one has a life-threatening disease; major changes in the routines of daily living; and the caregiver's assumption of the patient's household tasks. At the same time, many caregivers, particularly spouses or partners, can no longer turn to their own primary source of support—namely, the person who has cancer.

Issues

Caregivers often feel isolated and lonely, since extended family, friends, and health care providers are focusing all their attention on the patient. They may experience guilt as they become aware of their own needs, and tell themselves that these needs pale in comparison to those of the patient. You may hear caregivers remark, "I like it when someone asks how I'm doing as well as how

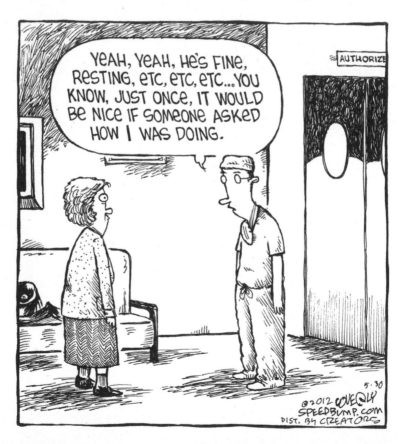

my wife is doing . . . I know it's really hard for her right now, but it is for me, too, although I can't complain; it seems so selfish and petty compared to her battle with cancer."

How can you help? Be on the alert for any clues caregivers may give, indicating what they need *right now*. (Caregivers' needs, like those of patients, will change over time.[1]) To support friends who are primary caregivers during cancer, keep the following six guidelines in mind:

1. **Acknowledge the fact that this experience affects the caregiver almost as much as the person with cancer.** Even when the caregiver denies the importance of his or her own needs, point out "how difficult this experience has to be for you as a caregiver," and offer opportunities for the caregiver to talk about his or her own feelings and thoughts.

2. **Keep your relationship much the same as it was before the loved one's diagnosis.** For example, if you and the caregiver enjoyed attending sporting events together, continue to suggest attending these, but recognize that the caregiver may not be as available. Consider changing how you spend time together—perhaps bringing a movie to the house and watching it with your friend instead of going to the theater. Remember, *the worst thing you can do is avoid caregiving friends*—even if you feel you are helping by not placing additional demands on their time.

3. **Recognize that sometimes the caregiver will want to keep cancer in the background.** We know that cancer survivors fluctuate between keeping cancer in the foreground and pushing it into the background to make life seem normal.[2] The same is true of caregivers. Sometimes what a caregiver

---

[1] Take a moment to skim chapters one through four again, this time keeping the *caregiver* in mind. Since caregivers approach their situations uniquely—with different needs at different times—pay particular attention to the section "Evaluate the Situation" in chapter one.

[2] Paterson, B. L. (2001). The shifting perspectives model of chronic illness. *Journal of Nursing Scholarship, 33*(1), 21-26.

wants is to talk about *anything but* cancer. It may help to ignore the cancer experience, even for a little while, especially when the experience feels too threatening, or when caregivers need a break.

4. **Remember that one of the hardest things to do is to ask for help.** Most caregivers believe they need to do what needs to be done *without complaint*. Many also feel they need to do it all, even when they are overwhelmed. Offer help with something specific on a day when the caregiver has many other things to do or when he or she needs to take some personal time. Even if your offer is not accepted at first, offer again at a later date. The caregiver may need to hear your offer several times before accepting it.

5. **Help caregivers recognize that reciprocity isn't always immediate or mutual.** Often people feel they must be able to reciprocate if someone helps them. Caregivers may be reluctant to accept help because they can't see how they would repay such help. Remind your caregiver-friend that being able to help at this time is rewarding in itself for you. Most people who want to help don't keep score or expect repayment. In the book *Pay It Forward*, author Catherine Ryan Hyde popularized the idea of asking that a good turn be repaid by doing something for *another* person—not the person who originally provided help or support. This is especially true during and after cancer.

6. **Encourage caregivers to stay healthy.** If caregivers aren't able to maintain their own emotional and physical health, they won't be able to continue to support patient-survivors. Part of staying healthy is taking time off for activities like hobbies or exercising. Friends can step in to provide caregiving relief by offering companionship or assistance directly to the patient, while at the same time encouraging the caregiver to take this time away for pleasurable activities—guilt-free!

Respite Care: The Wedding Trip

The waiting room was crowded as Gail reached for a magazine and Jim fidgeted anxiously. Both were short on patience. Gail couldn't help thinking of all she'd left undone. There were medical bills to pay, insurance forms to sort through, housekeeping, and yard work. Futhermore, Gail couldn't leave Jim alone long enough to grocery shop without worrying, "What if he falls while I'm gone? He can't even get to the phone."

The door opened and a pleasant voice interrupted their thoughts. "I have good news for you. Jim's condition has stabilized." Dr. Miller smiled warmly.

As they entered the examining room, Gail breathed a sigh of relief while Jim got ready for his check-up.

Dr. Miller quickly finished the exam. "You're looking good," she said, "and I'll see you back in a month."

When they stepped out into the hallway, Dr. Miller put a hand on Gail's arm and asked,

"Now that we know how Jim is doing, *how are you doing with Jim?*"

Gail's reserve crumbled and tears welled up in her eyes. "I'm running as fast as I can, but I just can't keep up," she said, a bit embarrassed.

Dr. Miller looked at her kindly. "I think you could use some help—perhaps some respite care?"

Gail nodded with her head down and left without saying a word.

On the ride home, Gail's thoughts turned to a difficult phone call she would make that afternoon. She and Jim couldn't attend their niece's wedding. He couldn't handle the flight from Phoenix to Indianapolis, much less negotiate stairs at their children's home once they arrived.

Gayle was about to have her own pity party when she remembered Dr. Miller's advice: *You need some help—perhaps respite care?* Where could she find facilities available for short-term *respite care*—care for people whose caregivers need a break?

When they arrived home, Gail decided to start by phoning the parish nurse at her church. The nurse told her that there were several options right in her own community; some provided care for just a few days and one for up to two weeks. Gail approached Jim tentatively. She held out the cream colored envelope containing the engraved wedding invitation. "Would you consider trying respite care just for a week, so I could go to the wedding with the kids?"

Jim grimaced. "All right," he said. He knew this was important to Gail.

Six weeks later Jim settled tentatively into a sunny, furnished room at Sedona Villa. For the next week, the Villa staff would provide Jim with meals and daily care as well as administer all his medications. "If a problem arises," the staff said, "we'll contact Dr. Miller, directly."

With a kiss and a catch in her breath—plus the promise of a nightly phone call—Gail waved good-bye to Jim and headed for her flight to Indianapolis.

While Gail was away, Jim admitted to having some trouble dealing with so many new people, but overall, he managed well. He said it felt good to be able to give Gail time with their family.

Gail returned energized and enthusiastic. "I feel as though I've been gone for a month. This was just what I needed," she said.

This totally new experience gave each of them something unexpected—a newfound sense of security. Now Gail and Jim knew that if respite care was ever needed again, it was available, affordable, and doable.

—*B.*

A Note on Respite Care: The American Cancer Society defines **respite care** as "short-term, temporary relief to those who are caring for family members who might otherwise need professional aid." ACS notes respite care can take place in patients' homes or in specialized facilities. They also advise that Medicare may assist with the costs (state-by-state) and that some health insurances may also help with respite care costs.

* American Cancer Society. *"What You Need to Know as a Cancer Caregiver"* last reviewed February 7, 2011, accessed February 25, 2012. (http://www.cancer. org/treatment/caregivers/index.)

TALKING TO CHILDREN ABOUT CANCER

Mother's Day

I remember the day as if it were yesterday. It was Mother's Day, 2002, and I was preparing to deliver the children's sermon. Twelve hours earlier the diagnosis had been confirmed—breast cancer—treatable, even curable, with extensive surgery and chemo. I typed and retyped the words until dawn. The children needed to hear the news first-hand rather than worry over whispers. Now it was time. . .

As the children tumbled out of the pews and came forward, we chatted about Mother's Day. I held up a four-generation photo and showed them my granddaughter Abby (three months), Beth (our daughter-in-law), and myself. Finally, I pointed out my seventy-nine-year old mother.

"This is my mom. A long time ago she was very, very sick. She went to the hospital, and after a while, she became very, very well. And now she is Baby Abby's Great-Grandma. Last night, I found out that I have the same sickness my mom had. And for a time I'm going to be very, very sick. I'll go to the hospital and after a while I hope to be very, very well too. Then, when Abby grows up and is the mommy, I can be the great-grandma too . . ."

After worship, the children responded predictably. Resilient and hopeful, they gave me hugs and kind words, saying they were sorry I was sick, and then moved immediately on to the important things of childhood—laughing, playing, and growing.

—B.

Another challenging situation is talking to children about cancer. What should we tell the kids? How do we reassure children who have a parent with cancer? Michelle Y. Pearlman, PhD, is a psychologist who was instrumental in helping New York City children understand and cope with the traumas of 9/11. She was the founding director of the Trauma and Bereavement Service at the NYU Child Study Center and is currently in private practice in New York and New Jersey.

WHAT TO SAY TO THE KIDS

by Michelle Pearlman, PhD

Adults commonly think that talking to children about illness and other potentially frightening topics will increase their anxiety, but this is not necessarily the case. Like adults, children's worries tend to increase when they are accompanied by uncertainty and confusion. When cancer is present, the most helpful thing is to engage children in an open discussion, dispel the confusion, and provide them with as much information as is appropriate for their ages and the given situation. The following guidelines may be helpful when speaking with children about cancer and related issues:

1. **Base the amount of information you share on the child's age, temperament, and interest.** In these conversations, it is usually helpful to explore what children think and understand. You might ask, "When you visited Mommy in the hospital, what did you see?" or "Is there anything you'd like to know about Mommy's sickness?"

   Follow the child's lead—continue to talk and provide answers as long as the child is interested, and allow the conversation to end (for the time being) when the child seems satisfied that his or her questions have been answered.

Out of the Mouths of Babes

Lois was diagnosed with breast cancer when her granddaughter, Liz, was just three years old. After several chemotherapy sessions, Lois's hair thinned and eventually fell out. She used bright scarves and a cute salt-and-pepper wig to camouflage her baldness. But children have a way of seeing past our best intentions to shield them from the truth. Liz was no exception; she was well aware Grandma Lois was sick with something called "cancer" and that she was bald.

The holidays were approaching, and Liz's mother called her into the kitchen. They sat down for a chat.

"Elizabeth, Grandma Lois is coming for a holiday visit," she said. Liz began bouncing up and down with excitement.

"But I want you to remember that Grandma has breast cancer and when she's here, she will need a little extra rest," said Mom.

Without skipping a beat Liz fired back, "Breast cancer? Oh, Mom, don't be silly. Grandma Lois doesn't have breast cancer. She has hair cancer!"

—B

2. **Provide children with honest and direct information about the illness.** We build and maintain trust by being truthful with children. Choose clear language to describe the illness and related medical procedures. For example, concrete terms should be used to prepare children for what they might see. "You will see a little machine on wheels that gives Mommy medicine right through a special tube in her arm." A brief explanation can also help children know what they might expect over time. "Every two weeks, Daddy will need to go back to the clinic during the day for chemotherapy treatments, but he'll be home before supper."

3. **Encourage children to share their thoughts and feelings—confusion, worry, anger, or sadness—with a parent or another adult.** Some children may want to talk about what is happening, while others may prefer to express themselves through art or by connecting with peers.

4. **It is important *not* to judge one child's reactions by another's.** Some children will find solace by spending time with friends and relatives, while others will prefer to process the difficult news on their own. Reassure the child that it is normal to experience many different reactions to stress (including anger, guilt, and sadness), and that a person may feel sadness without necessarily crying.

5. **Allow children to retain as much of their daily routines as possible during stressful times.** By maintaining familiar schedules, children will gradually reestablish feelings of normalcy, and their anxieties will be significantly reduced.

6. **Every child will process information at his/her own pace.** Be available to discuss the illness on more than one occasion, since children's questions and interest in the situation will change over time.

7. **Mood changes are to be expected in children in response to upsetting events.** Be aware of (and patient with) these possible fluctuations in a child's emotions. Reassure

patients' children that no matter what happens, they will always be loved and cared for.

8. **Provide children with choices about their level of involvement.** Children should not be forced to visit loved ones in the hospital, but the option should be available for those who express interest. Provide options to help children maintain connections and demonstrate their care by creating cards or gifts and making phone calls.

If adults avoid discussions about potentially worrisome situations, they may convey to children that the topic is "taboo"; this may ultimately result in increasing children's fears and worry. Instead, find words and ways to share the truth with children in an honest yet hopeful manner.[3]

WHEN THE PATIENT IS A CHILD

When we think of cancer, we often picture a middle-aged grandparent or empty-nesters. Another set of special situations arises when cancer occurs at other times in the life cycle—such as in childhood or adolescence. The following three sections will help you understand the challenges and unique issues that confront patients and their families when the patient is a child, a teen, or an older adult.

Linda White is an accomplished music educator and composer. Linda and I have been best friends for over thirty years. In 2007 she was named to the National Teacher's Hall of Fame, *USA Today's* "All USA Teacher Team," and was Virginia's Outstanding General Music Educator. Linda's biggest challenge and accomplishment, however, was not in the field of education. It was helping her young son and her family survive his experience of

---

[3] Dr. Wendy Schlessel Harpham, MD, has written a very helpful book on this topic for all adults, *When a Parent Has Cancer: A Guide to Caring for Your Children.* Dr. Harpham says, "When the facts are couched in love and hopefulness, you can guide your children toward a life-enhancing perception of reality." (New York: Perennial Currents, 2004), 8. First published by Harper-Collins Publishers in 1997.

pediatric cancer.[4] I spoke with Linda and her adult daughter, Meg, about their experiences.

PEDIATRIC CANCER: A CONVERSATION

Bonnie: What are the issues that parents face when one of their children has cancer?

Linda: As in most cancer situations, there are so many "what ifs." What if your child doesn't make it? What if the money runs out? What if you can't make it home from the hospital to meet the school bus carrying your other children? You can't plan anything. Everything feels out of control.

Furthermore, when your child is diagnosed with cancer, you use up all of your energy becoming this child's advocate. Even when you try your best, you feel that what you are doing is never enough. This leaves little or no energy to nurture other relationships. You know you are short-changing your spouse and your other children, but you are trying to keep this child alive. Everyone in the family is being impacted by this experience.

Bonnie: Meg, you were pretty young when your brother had cancer. Tell us how cancer impacts siblings.

Meg: I was only eight years old when my brother was diagnosed with cancer, so I often felt left out. I found it difficult to relate to kids my age that didn't have a sick sibling. My hair was braided by the neighbors; I ate hospital food instead of meals at home; and a neighbor met my school bus instead of my mom. It was hard!

Naturally, my brother received all kinds of gifts, bears, and toys, and as a child, I wondered, *where are my new toys?* Everyone who came to the hospital was so excited to see him—what about me? In looking back, it seems one of the most important things friends can do is to remember the siblings. Whenever you bring something for the patient, remember to bring something for other children in the family.

---

[4]   Linda and Bill White's son, Matthew, was diagnosed with stage four pediatric kidney cancer (Wilm's Tumor) when he was just six years old. Matt underwent over a year and a half of treatments. Recently married, Matt is a long-term cancer survivor and college graduate who lives and works in the Washington, DC area.

Additionally, brothers and sisters of pediatric patients often sense that the entire universe revolves around the sick child; their own identities can easily become tied up with the ill child. Siblings need to feel they are valued as independent beings with identities all their own.

When visiting, take time to talk with siblings and ask them questions that have nothing to do with the sick child—questions about *their* interests or hobbies. Make plans to spend special time with siblings; they need to anticipate activities and events that are not tied to the patient's health, whether that means going to a movie with an auntie or looking forward to an ice-skating date with a classmate.

Finally, the concept of "future" is nebulous for children; I often wondered if the future meant I would always have a brother with cancer. Do some research for families facing cancer and help to find venues where siblings of cancer patients can network with each other and share their common experiences.[5]

Bonnie: **What are some examples of ways friends can help out during pediatric cancer?**

Linda: As the parent of a child with cancer, all your emotions reside just beneath the surface—the tears, the anger, the guilt, the fear of how it will all turn out. There were some days I just wanted to go into a corner and cry. Often I couldn't leave the hospital, so I especially appreciated friends who came to just sit quietly with me and friends who dropped by saying, "We've come to bring you lunch!" These friends gave me space to talk or be silent, to vent, or even cry. As with other cancer situations, this was a time for my friends to listen; NOT to criticize, NOT to offer advice—just to *be there*!

On the practical side, gas cards, grocery cards (so friends could stock the fridge), and people to do the laundry were particularly helpful. I often joke that my spouse's underwear was folded by more women in Florida than anyone else's.

---

[5] There are many camps for pediatric patients and/or siblings of seriously ill children, as well as local cancer family support groups. The Children's Oncology Camping Association-International (COCA-I) lists over sixty-five member camps in the United States alone, as well as a number of international camps.

Parents of pediatric patients need friends who are available for last minute requests—friends who don't mind hearing, "Matt hasn't been eating and suddenly today he's hungry for _____. Could you run over to get some and bring it to the hospital?"

Friends who *directly* help out the patient's family, *indirectly* give ill children more time to spend with their parents. Enabling parents to stay in close proximity to hospitalized children is a gift to both of them. You can research local Ronald McDonald houses or area churches/mosques/synagogues that may be willing to assist parents living away from home. You can also ask the cancer care center if they have a list of nearby accommodations or if they provide social workers to help families. Remember, cancer or no cancer, pediatric patients are first and foremost kids. They may not feel up to regular activities on some days, but on others they work through the pain to enjoy things children love—fishing off the hospital pier, pigging out on hot dogs or powdered sugar doughnuts, or just playing with their favorite toys.

Modern technology also enables hospitalized or homebound students to Skype with friends and classmates. Many young patients have access to iPads or laptops; if not, schools or friends can pool resources to provide them for the patient and his/her family. Young patients and their families may also request that someone act as a liaison with the school, e.g., pick up/deliver school assignments or keep in touch with teachers.

Finally, spend time with pediatric patients—reading or playing computer games, cards, and board games. (Check with the pediatric cancer center to see if healthy children can visit.) And remember when you send gifts to pediatric cancer patients, it is in the child's best interest to space out gifts and not to over-do. Instead, try sending a package of smaller gifts for parents to distribute at appropriate times, rather than one over-the-top gift.

No matter what you choose to do, or how you choose to help, always remember that cancer impacts an entire family, not just the pediatric patient. The whole family benefits when friends nurture *each and every family member.*

TEENS AND YOUNG ADULTS

At least two hundred and seventy thousand of today's cancer survivors were diagnosed before the age of twenty-one.[6] Amy Blumenfeld[7] is the voice of young-adult cancer survivorship. She is an accomplished journalist and childhood-cancer survivor who gives us a personal and candid perspective on the unique cancer challenges faced by teens and young adults. She also discusses how you can help them.

Cancer as a Teen or Young Adult

by Amy Blumenfeld, MS

Friendship is particularly precious for teens and young adults battling disease during the formative years of their lives. Pre-teen years and adolescence are challenging years for everyone. It's an awkward time when our bodies grow and rebel with pimples, growth spurts, and vocal chord changes. When that same body wages a war against itself even further by developing cancer in the midst of puberty, it's asking a lot physically. To lose your hair from chemo when you're ready for your first kiss—and to know you need Mom and Dad's assistance with the most personal of tasks while simultaneously attempting to establish your independence—is asking a lot emotionally. To conquer the disease and emerge from it all as a healthy, productive person, and fade into society with few physical scars, is simply a miracle.

Unlike adult patients who have lived several decades as healthy, productive individuals, these kids are in the midst of growing up when first diagnosed and treated.

The Issues

Everyone with cancer has concerns no matter what their age—the possibility of relapse, fear of the unknown, and acceptance

---

[6] National Cancer Institute, "The Childhood Cancer Survivor Study: An Overview," originally posted 01/10/2007, updated 06/06/2012. www.cancer.gov/cancertopics/coping/ccss.

[7] © Amy Blumenfeld, All Rights Reserved, 2012. Used by permission.

by peers both socially and professionally. Teen and young adult patients also have unique concerns.

People like me don't wonder in our 50's if our husbands will find us attractive post-mastectomy or if we will have the stamina to run around with our grandchildren after a dose of chemo. Instead, we pray as eighth graders that the drugs and radiation we have received will not only spare our lives, but our fertility as well— even at an age when the concept of having our own children is virtually impossible to grasp.

Later on, we fear rejection from a potential spouse once we disclose not only our history of illness, but also the possibility that we may never be able to conceive. Will we be branded as damaged goods? And if that is a potential reaction, should we disclose our illness at the start of a relationship, or wait, only to risk losing someone we have grown to love?

Furthermore, how will cancer impact our careers? Adult patients and survivors have had years to establish themselves professionally. As teens and young adults, we are just starting out. If our first employer is informed of our recent battle, will we be rejected because of a concern we may relapse on the job, or will our status as a "fighter" and "survivor" work to our advantage?

The issues facing those of us who struggle with cancer before adulthood are many. Here is a sampling of our concerns, the issues we face, and how you can help:

Hair Loss

Hair loss is traumatic at any age, but can be particularly challenging during adolescence—a time fraught with insecurity. In fact, it's not unusual for some children and teens to have a greater fear of hair loss than death. In the minds of teens, kids are immortal; but hair loss is social death, particularly for girls. It is emotionally debilitating, alienating, and some are convinced that their appearance will scare away friends, not to mention potential partners. Others, however, find hair loss to be empowering. The crumbling of facades and being forced to confront the world as a pasty, follicularly-challenged teen can uncover a latent inner strength and the existence of an unknown steel.

As a friend, the most important message you can convey is: "I love you for what is on the inside, not the outside." How you express and drive home that message is up to you. Shave your head in solidarity? Shower her with funky scarves and him with baseball caps? Grow out your own hair to donate to an organization like Locks of Love that makes wigs for kids with cancer?[8] Go to a salon for makeovers and a day of beauty? Whatever you do, make it fun and be sure she knows you are by her side no matter how she looks.

New Family Dynamics

Another rite of passage often experienced by survivors of childhood and adolescent disease is changing relationships with parents and siblings. During illness, parents were the caretakers, and many needs of healthy siblings may have been temporarily placed on the back burner. Now that the patient (adolescent) is healthy, there is a new dynamic. Transitioning from a family in a cancer crisis to a family post-crisis is certainly welcome, but it comes with its share of growing pains.

For instance, during illness, there was likely a lack of physical privacy for patients—they were dependent on parents for even the most personal of tasks. Now, there are new boundaries that parents must respect. Healthy siblings may feel resentful. The patient may feel guilty for having "stolen" parents' attention. When treatment ends, every family shifts gears regardless of the issues. As a friend, you may be just the right person to hold the survivor's hand as she jumps these emotional and personal hurdles.

Disclosure and Relationships

How do you tell someone you have just started dating that you recently overcame a life-threatening illness, that it could relapse, that the treatment put you at higher risk for a secondary cancer, and that it might have left you infertile? The answer: Gracefully.

---

[8] Locks of Love is a public not-for-profit that creates hairpieces for children in need under twenty-one, who suffer long-term or permanent medical hair loss due to cancer and other medical conditions. Hairpieces are fashioned from donated hair (www. locksoflove.org).

There is no easy way for a young cancer survivor to disclose the long-term effects of his cancer treatment with a potential spouse. He'll hope for the best, but expect the worst. Survivors' minds are flooded with questions: Should I start the conversation early in the relationship to spare rejection later on when I have fallen in love? Or will doing so cause the other person to feel I am propelling the relationship forward at warp speed?

If you are a friend who is dating a young cancer survivor, don't feel guilty if you have reservations about entering into a serious relationship. Think everything through. Be honest with yourself and with your partner. Once you commit to being with a survivor long-term, you inherit all of their medical and emotional concerns, making you, in a sense, a side effect of their side effects. If the survivor has a weak immune system, it may impact everything from travel plans to everyday life. If the survivor is infertile or needs medical assistance in creating a family, there are physical, emotional, and financial matters that you should be aware of. If you marry the survivor, what happens if they don't qualify for life insurance because of their medical history?

Life is an unknown, especially in the world of cancer. As the significant other, ask yourself, "Am I emotionally prepared should cancer reappear? If need be, am I comfortable being a caretaker?" Most people will rise to the occasion, but if you find yourself becoming anxious just thinking about the possibility, you might want to speak with a medical professional. Having an expert answer some of your questions may help quell some of your fears. Also, there are plenty of support groups for partners—check with your local hospital or any national cancer organization for their local chapters.

Every year seventy-two thousand adolescents and young adults are diagnosed with cancer.[9] While their futures hold unanswered questions, their tenacity, courage, and resolve deserve our highest respect and serve as examples to all of us.

---

[9] Fifteen to thirty-nine years of age. Statistics from: "Adolescents and Young Adults with Cancer," National Cancer Institute. (www.cancer.gov, accessed 11/2/2011).

New Beginnings

by Amy Blumenfeld, MS

It wasn't until I started dating seriously that disclosure became an issue. In no way was I ashamed of my cancer history; in fact, there was an element of pride in having overcome a life-threatening disease at a young age. But I knew that even the greatest guy in the world would have reason to pause before marrying someone who could relapse, develop a secondary cancer, or be infertile.

By all accounts, my health and fertility were intact, but given that my treatment was intense and experimental, not even the most-renowned doctors could accurately predict the future.

In 2000, at the age of twenty-six, I found that great guy. His response was better than I had ever expected. He was interested in all aspects of my history; he was proud of what I had overcome, and when I told him I didn't know if we would be able to have a child, his response was, without skipping a beat, "So, we'll adopt." When we wed two years later, Dan knew he was marrying me as well as my survivorship—for better or worse.

A couple of years later, we learned that the high-dose radiation had damaged my uterus so severely that I am incapable of carrying a pregnancy to term. However, because my doctors had the foresight when I was fourteen years old to shift my ovaries out of the line of radiation and shield them, my eggs remained healthy and I was able to have my own biological child. With the help of in vitro fertilization, we created our own genetic embryo and transferred it to another woman's uterus. She became pregnant with our baby and, to our great joy delivered our daughter in February 2006.

Freedom

by Amy Blumenfeld, MS

I recall the day I was discharged from Memorial Sloan-Kettering, after nearly two months in a reverse isolation room for an autologous bone marrow transplant. I was escorted through the hospital doors and onto Manhattan's York Avenue, where I sat in a wheelchair awaiting my ride home. I inhaled the sweet summer air as deeply as I could. Even the thick black exhaust from the trucks merging onto the Queensboro Bridge smelled divine. It's amazing what regaining your freedom can do to your senses.

Yet, as I sat there, acutely aware of every possible germ source, I felt more restricted than ever before. It was as if anything contagious had been highlighted. I envisioned dancing amoebae on taxi door handles. I squirmed when a child walking by coughed without covering his mouth. And upon hearing a sneeze, my eyes instantly darted to pinpoint its exact location.

Before discharge, doctors explained that the chemo and radiation had weakened my immunity to the point that I was highly susceptible to nearly any bug out there. Certain places, such as enclosed spaces without much fresh air, were off limits. No movie theaters. No restaurants. No public transportation. No mall. And it's a good thing I didn't like sushi because uncooked food was a thing of the past, at least for the time being. It was as if I was handed an instruction manual for freedom.

Fortunately, my friends and family were incredibly supportive. No pity. No coddling. Humor infused everything possible. They aimed to make recovery fun—a group project. We played highly competitive games of Scrabble in my parents' den. Our next-door neighbors cooked delicious authentic Italian meals they swore would boost my immune system. My cousins sent a garbage bag full of Max Factor make-up so I could be the hottest bald fifteen-year-old girl in town. We baked cookies, rented movies, and our neighborhood walks lengthened as the weeks passed.

"It takes a village to raise a child," and I believe it can easily translate to healing a patient. My doctors drew up the battle plan and created the strategy, but my family and friends helped me fight and win.

CANCER IN OLDER ADULTS

The likelihood of developing cancer increases with age. Nearly 30 percent of all cancers are diagnosed in people seventy-five years or older.[10] This is a unique group of patients who are dealing with multiple health issues beyond cancer. In seeking expertise on cancer in older adults, I turned to Rev. Gloria Steadman-Sannermark, a registered nurse and clergywoman. Rev. Sannermark has been a hospice chaplain and currently ministers to older adults in the Sun Cities of Arizona.

When the Patient is Older

by Rev. Gloria Steadman-Sannermark, RN, MDiv

Two characteristics stand out when I observe older adults with cancer—attitude and overload. A fellow clergyman, Rev. Tim Smith, puts it this way, "Older adults have been through life's trials and tend to take the news [of cancer] with a *go-ahead-and-tell-me-attitude....* They don't want to suffer, but they are not afraid to die."[11]

---

[10] SEER Cancer Statistics Review, 1975-2009 (Vintage 2009 Populations), "Table 1.10. Age Distribution (%) of Incidence Cases by Site, 2005–2009," National Cancer Institute, http://seer.cancer.gov/csr/1975_2009_pops09/.

[11] Rev. Tim Smith in an interview with Gloria Steadman-Sannermark (Phoenix, Arizona, 2006).

A diagnosis of cancer affirms what older adults already know—life on this earth is finite, and living is not measured in time, but in quality of life.

Older adults are overwhelmed and overloaded. They are dealing with cancer at the same time that they are confronting many other losses. These include the loss of friends, of health, of mobility, and of independence. The impact and significance of these age-related losses is easily overlooked. "It's as if age somehow [makes these] losses less meaningful," says Rev. Smith.[12]

Older adults also face special challenges that accompany changing times. In the past, adults accepted medical authority without question. Now older adults find it expected—even necessary—to challenge medical opinions. Many are uncomfortable even collaborating with their physicians in decision-making regarding their treatments or care. They also fear the prospect of spending time in a nursing home or other health care facility, and wonder where they'll find the resources to pay for such care. They worry about making sense of the paperwork generated by mounting medical bills and insurance claims, and they struggle to maintain long-held values of privacy, independence, and personal control over finances and other private information.

However, if you have older friends with cancer, don't assume they are needy just because of advancing age. *Being elderly is more a state of mind than a chronological age.* Even those without close family are creative in orchestrating their cancer care and meeting their own special needs. Furthermore, many older adults are computer savvy or adept at finding needed information. Even with countless challenges, many older adults survive cancer multiple times, struggle with other age-related illnesses, and still continue to live meaningful, enjoyable, and active lives. They focus on quality of life and often are less concerned about themselves than about those they might leave behind.

---

[12] Ibid.

Maxine and Peter

Maxine and Peter were members of my congregation. College sweethearts, their lives diverged following graduation. Both married others, raised families, retired, and lost their spouses. When Maxine learned that Peter's wife had died, she sent him a sympathy card with her return address. Knowing time was precious, Peter wasted little in tracking down Maxine. He flew across the country and vowed not to return home without her.

The two married, and a scant two months later, Maxine was diagnosed with breast cancer. "I wasn't afraid to die, but I didn't want to leave him. Peter's love held me," she said. After Peter nursed her back to health, Maxine cared for him until his death from cancer, years later.

At her ninetieth birthday celebration, Maxine rejoiced even in the face of her loss. She said, "We had sixteen years together; the best sixteen years of our lives!"

by Rev. Gloria Steadman-Sannermark

For some, cancer will be their final struggle. In this case, you may be the one trusted friend who is able to walk alongside a patient-friend through the closures and good-byes. To do this, listen to an older friend's fears and triumphs. Be willing to circumvent the polite small talk, hear the hard stuff, and let your patient-friend address meaningful issues which might be upsetting to other family members or friends.

In most cases, older adults know the implications of their illness (especially when cancer is life-threatening) and they know that *you* know! Good friends allow them the opportunities to say what they need to say without having to be brave for others.

Helping Out

by Rev. Gloria Steadman-Sannermark, RN, MDiv

How can you provide meaningful support and an improved quality of life for older friends? Here are several questions to help you evaluate your older friend's needs and wishes:

1. **Has cancer overshadowed necessary attention to your friend's multiple health concerns?** Offer to pick up medications, provide transportation to the doctor, or even schedule necessary appointments, if needed.

2. **Does your older friend need a health care advocate or insurance advocate?** If you know your way around Medicare and health plans, offer assistance when insurance claims seem overwhelming.

3. **Does your friend need help with a dependent spouse, sibling, or even a parent?** Ask if you might look in on a dependent spouse or parent when your friend is ill or hospitalized. (There also may be pet at home that needs looking after.)

4. **Watch for signs of depression,** such as sleeplessness, not eating, or lack of personal care. Depression is common in older adults with multiple health concerns or losses and can be deepened by the news of cancer. As a friend, remember that listening can be one of the very best antidotes for depression; however, depression can be a serious condition and medical or psychological counseling may be warranted when the above signs are present.

5. **Ask if anyone has been in touch with your friend's religious community.** Many in the senior population regard church, synagogue, or mosque as the defining community in which they are known. Offer to be a contact person to relay information that your

patient-friend would like to share with clergy, the parish nurse, or the community at large.

6. **Inquire about caregiver(s).** Take note of your friend's spouse or caregiver. Is he or she rested, in good spirits and, healthy?

7. **If long-term homecare or self-care appears difficult, help older adults research other residential options.** A variety of facilities and residences offer special amenities such as on-site nursing, meal plans, vans, and assisted or independent living. Encourage your friend to explore residential options earlier rather than later. This provides an opportunity to make a new residence "home," and solves many housekeeping and meal preparation issues during and after cancer.

8. **Ask, "What would make your life *most meaningful now?*"** A meaningful quality of life for an older adult may mean finding a way to achieve a lifelong dream, reunite a family, or simply attend a major-league ball game and get on with life in spite of cancer. Ask if you can help your friend make special plans or achieve a long-held goal.

9. **Help your older friend make a "File for Life" to keep information for future decision-making.** Include information on agencies providing home-health care assistance, brochures received during visits to care or assisted living facilities, and his or her preferences regarding hospice care (if needed). Encourage your friend to tell family members where this file is kept.

Chapter Seven

ASK THE EXPERTS: CANCER Q&A WHAT FRIENDS SHOULD KNOW

CANCER 101

When you want to know more about cancer and its treatments, it is time to consult the experts. Misinformation fuels fear. In this chapter, cancer professionals will answer the most common questions about cancer treatments and procedures. (See the footnote below regarding additional treatment options.[1])

We begin with two New York doctors, Melissa Gill, MD, and Anjali Saqi, MD. Dr. Gill is a pathologist who devotes much of her time to collaborative research in dermatology and dermatopathology. She is the founder and medical director of SkinMedical Research and Diagnostics. Dr. Saqi is associate professor of Pathology and Cell biology at New York Presbyterian Hospital,

---

[1] This chapter discusses the most common cancer treatments. There are other treatment approaches and therapies, including some in clinical trials. Information on additional treatment approaches and therapies may be found by accessing the website: www.cancer.gov. There you will find information on: angiogenesis, biological therapy, bone marrow transplantation, gene therapy, hyperthermia therapy, laser therapy, photodynamic therapy, targeted therapy and more. These treatments/therapies are briefly defined in this book's glossary.

Columbia University Medical Center. They will help us understand what it means when a friend says, "I need a biopsy."

BIOPSIES

What Friends Want to Know
by Melissa Gill, MD, and Anjali Saqi, MD, MBA

What are biopsies?
A biopsy is a small sample of cells or tissue fragment(s) obtained from anywhere in the body, intended for examination by pathologists using a microscope. Biopsies are performed to diagnose both **cancerous** and **benign** lesions (abnormal tissue). Because biopsies are small samples, occasionally the initial sample is not sufficient to make an adequate diagnosis. In such instances, a repeat biopsy may be necessary.

Is there more than one kind of biopsy?
Yes. A **fine needle aspiration** (FNA) uses a thin needle, placed briefly in the lesion to obtain a sample of cells. A **needle core biopsy** uses a larger needle to obtain a sample of solid tissue rather than cells. This biopsy is generally done under local anesthesia. Both may be repeated a few times to ensure that enough tissue is obtained. **Excisional biopsies** may be performed in a doctor's office (if the lesion is superficial) or in the operating room. In certain circumstances, such as breast, thyroid, or some soft tissue lesions, excisional biopsy may be performed after an earlier diagnosis has been made by FNA and/or needle-core biopsy. There are also specialized biopsies, including **shave biopsy, and punch biopsy** (usually used for skin lesions), and **sentinel lymph node biopsy.**

Are biopsies needed for definitive cancer diagnosis?
Yes. The gold standard for diagnosis of cancer is examination of the tissue by light microscopy. This biopsy diagnosis of cancer is usually necessary prior to surgery, although a strong clinical or radiographical suspicion is also sufficient.

How soon will my friend know the results of his or her biopsy?

Reassure your patient-friend that a longer wait for results does not mean cancer is present! Biopsy results are usually available within a few days to a week following the procedure. Finally, if there is ever a concern, one can always get a second pathology opinion on the biopsy.

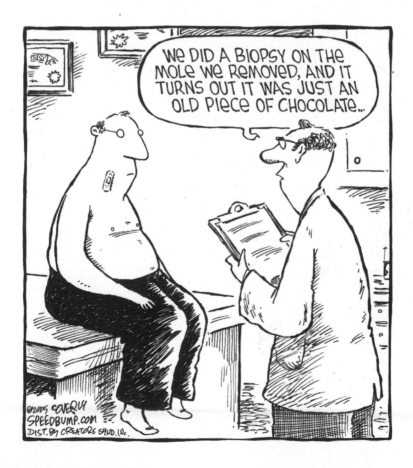

CANCER SURGERY

When a biopsy has confirmed the presence of cancer, one of the first questions patients ask is, "Will I need surgery?" Heather Richardson, MD, a general surgeon practicing in Atlanta, Georgia, helps us understand when surgery is needed and answers our basic questions about cancer surgery.

What Friends Want to Know

by Heather Richardson, MD

Is surgery necessary for all cancers?

No, not always. Surgery is the treatment choice for cancers that appear to be concentrated in one area. Other treatments are typically favored over surgery if the risk of damage to important surrounding healthy tissues outweighs the benefit from the removal of the cancer. Cancers that appear in many places in the body at once, such as lymphoma or leukemia, are not usually treated primarily with surgery.

Most patients will need a surgical procedure at some point during their cancer journey. Surgery may be used to obtain tissue for diagnosis (e.g., excisional or sentinel node biopsies). Surgical procedures are also used to insert and remove devices that permit chemotherapy to be infused (ports), and of course, for the removal of the cancer itself.

My friend just wants the cancer *out*. Is there time to consider a second opinion?

Patients often feel a sense of urgency and want to begin treatment as soon as possible. They do not realize that *the speed at which cancers grow and develop varies*. Most cancers develop slowly enough for thorough plans to be made and choices reviewed. Today, many cancers are caught at a stage where options can be investigated and patients have time to seek second opinions.

If your friend's cancer diagnosis was made because of symptoms of pain, organ dysfunction, intestinal blockage, or neurological change, surgical intervention becomes *much more urgent.* Even if the patient is symptom free, *some cancers progress rapidly,* and beginning treatment as soon as possible gives your friend a greater chance of cure or a decreased chance of problems.

How will my friend know if the surgery has been successful?
Even in a seemingly routine surgery, there is no way to tell whether or not all cancer has been eradicated at the time of the surgery. The goal is to see that the cancer is well contained within the tissue removed. This is often described as "having clear margins."

The most important indicator of whether a surgery was successful is the information from the tissue analysis or pathology report. The spread of cancer to lymph nodes implies that the cancer can leave the site of origin, and this affects your friend's prognosis. It does not mean cure is impossible, but that tiny cells may have drifted away from the site of the cancer's origin.

How can my friend find a good surgeon?
Confidence in, and good communication with, the surgeon are very important. Obviously, the more often a surgeon has treated your friend's particular problem, the better; someone who has regular experience with the problem is ideal. It is also important to work with a surgeon who is board certified in his or her area of practice.

If your friend's problem is a rare one, if the treatment recommendations are risky, or if the overall prognosis is poor, it may be a good idea to contact a cancer center that is conducting research in that area, or a center with specialists who have more experience with uncommon diseases or presentations.

RECONSTRUCTIVE SURGERY

When patients require or request reconstructive procedures following cancer surgery, new questions arise. Joseph Disa, MD, a well-known plastic surgeon, and Danielle Ferrer, RN, address these questions. Both work at Memorial Sloan-Kettering Cancer Center in New York City. Dr. Disa is the author of *100 Questions and Answers about Breast Surgery.*

What Friends Want to Know

by Danielle Ferrer, RN, and Joseph J. Disa, MD

What are some of the reasons my friend may select or require reconstructive surgery?

If the cancer surgeon is unable to close a wound after removing a tumor, reconstruction may be necessary to cover the surgical defect. Reconstruction is also done to aid or improve function (for example, to help with chewing, swallowing, walking, etc.) or to improve a patient's appearance. Reconstruction can help restore or improve a person's body image, which may have been altered by surgical treatment. Reconstruction can also help a patient return to normal activities, and it can improve a patient's quality of life.

What are the types of reconstructive surgery and when do they take place?

The most common cancer reconstructive surgery for women is breast reconstruction following mastectomy. This can be done either at the time of mastectomy or at a later date. Breast reconstruction can be accomplished with either an implant-based reconstruction or by "borrowing" tissue from another part of the body.

A common type of cancer reconstructive surgery for men is head-and-neck reconstruction following surgery to remove cancer in these areas. For example, jaw-bone (mandible) reconstruction is commonly accomplished by "borrowing" a bone and other tissue, as needed, from the lower leg. Reconstruction can occur anywhere on the body.

Sometimes reconstruction is performed at the time of the cancer removal and sometimes at a later date. Reconstruction of certain areas (head and neck, chest, abdomen, pelvis, or extremities) is almost always done at the time of tumor removal to avoid serious and potentially life-threatening complications. There are choices in the timing of breast reconstruction, and your patient-friend should ask her doctor whether immediate or delayed breast reconstruction is a better choice for her.

How should my friend choose a reconstructive surgeon?
Your friend should consult with a surgeon who is board-certified.[2]
Reconstructive surgeons typically are plastic surgeons and have
been certified by the American Board of Plastic Surgery. You
can confirm that a physician is board certified on websites such
as the American Board of Medical Specialties at www.abms.
org or the American Board of Plastic Surgery at www.abplsurg.
org. In addition to checking on board certification, it is a good
idea to research a surgeon's experience with your friend's particular type of reconstruction. It is also important for your
patient-friend to feel comfortable with, and confident in, his or
her chosen health care provider.

How might my friend feel after reconstructive surgery?
After any surgery, post-operative discomfort can be expected at
the surgical site(s). The level of pain can vary from very mild to
severe, and it tends to decrease with the passing of time. Someone
who is undergoing major abdominal surgery, for example, can
expect more discomfort than someone undergoing closure of a
small facial wound after removal of a skin cancer. Your friend may
also have various tubes, such as drains or catheters, after surgery,
and while they may be cumbersome, most of these are not painful.

Problems: When to take your friend back to the doctor.
Your friend or his/her care partner should contact the doctor with
any concerns. Before going home from the hospital, a patient is
typically given a written list of conditions that definitely warrant
a phone call or trip to the doctor. This will usually include
signs or symptoms of infection—such as a fever, chills, redness
at the surgical site, increased pain, or a foul-smelling drainage
from the surgical incision or wound. Also, commonly included
are problems such as bleeding, nausea/vomiting, and diarrhea.
There may also be specific things to watch for, depending on the
type and/or location of surgery; the surgeon and other members

---

[2] Certification by the American Board of Medical Specialties requires the doctor to have
completed training in an accredited institution and to have successfully passed any
requisite examinations for the specialty.

of the health care team (resident, nurse, physician assistant, etc.) should tell your friend what to watch out for. Remember, if there is *any question or other concern*, your friend or his/her care partner should contact the doctor.

CHEMOTHERAPY

In considering possible cancer therapies, the question "Will he or she need chemotherapy?" invariably arises. Dr. Julie Monroe is a prominent suburban New York oncologist known for her compassionate care and her knowledge of the latest cancer treatments. For ten years she and I have traveled the cancer journey together as doctor and patient. Dr. Monroe and her colleague, Dr. Henry Lee, are my go-to doctors for information on the chemotherapy experience.

What Friends Want to Know

by Julie Monroe, MD, and Henry Lee, MD, PhD

What is chemotherapy?
Chemotherapy is the treatment of cancer with drugs that can destroy cancer cells. These anticancer drugs work by stopping cells from growing and multiplying. Since cancer cells tend to grow rapidly, they are susceptible to these drugs. Combination chemotherapy—the use of several drugs together—works by attacking the cancer cells at different critical points in their growth cycles, which makes the therapy more effective. This approach also reduces the chance that cancer cells will become resistant to drugs.

My friend is having "adjuvant" chemotherapy. What does this mean?
Chemotherapy can be given at different times during a patient's treatment course. **Adjuvant chemotherapy** is used to treat early stage cancer in an effort to eradicate any residual cancerous cell

which may have been left behind by surgery to cure the cancer and reduce the risk of a future relapse. **Neoadjuvant chemotherapy** is given before surgery often when the tumor is large in an effort to shrink the tumor to allow for a more adequate surgical resection. **Palliative chemotherapy** is used to treat more advanced disease in an effort to relieve symptoms (such as pain), improve quality of life, and possibly prolong survival.

How will my friend receive chemotherapy?

Different types of cancer are treated with different types of chemotherapy. Some chemotherapy drugs are administered by infusion (intravenous drips into the veins), others by injection (shots) or orally (pills). Treatments can usually be given in an outpatient setting such as a doctor's office or a hospital infusion center, but some treatments require an overnight stay at the hospital. Certain treatments are given over several hours in one day, while other regimens require several days.

Does everyone experience the same side effects from chemotherapies?

Healthy cells in the body can also be harmed by chemotherapy, especially those that divide quickly (such as those found in hair follicles, the gastrointestinal lining, and blood cells). It is this harm to healthy cells that causes the side effects of chemotherapy.

Side effects can be different, depending on which drugs your friend receives and/or how they are given. For instance, not all chemotherapy drugs cause hair loss. Certain drugs can either be given at a larger dose once every three weeks or at smaller doses weekly; side effects vary with the different schedules.

One of the most common side effects of chemotherapy is fatigue. Friends and loved ones undergoing chemotherapy may not be feeling up to doing everything they usually do and may need to take naps during the day. If a friend has a lot of side effects from chemotherapy, it does not mean his or her cancer-related prognosis is any better or worse than someone experiencing only a few. If a friend has minimal side effects or none at all, it does *not* mean that the treatments are not working.

Can chemotherapy be utilized more than once in treating cancer?
Sometimes chemotherapy initially works to control a cancer, but over time the cancer becomes resistant to that drug or combination of drugs. When a cancer becomes resistant to one chemotherapy drug, it may subsequently respond to a different chemotherapy drug or combination of drugs.

Don't Be Surprised If . . .

1. Your friend has good and bad days.
Energy levels fluctuate and responses to therapies (side effects) vary during a normal treatment cycle; some days are simply better than others. It often helps to ask, "Is today a good time to visit/talk/attend a meeting?" Be prepared to alter plans at a moment's notice.

2. Certain foods or smells are unwelcome.
Patients may order a favorite food only to find that it suddenly tastes or smells different. You can avoid some of these surprises by asking, "Do any particular foods or smells bother you?"

3. Your friend appears forgetful or unable to concentrate.
Even the most dependable friend or employee may forget an appointment or miss a deadline during treatment. During and after chemotherapy, however, many survivors report unanticipated memory and cognitive challenges.

New research has discovered the combination of certain chemotherapy drugs can result in long-term effects on a patient's cognitive processing. These side effects are called "chemo-brain" and are variously characterized by difficulties with word recall, multi-tasking, cognitive processing, and even manual dexterity. While many patients recover these cognitive skills within one to five years, one study found patients still suffering from lingering cognitive difficulties decades later. It is unknown whether these effects might be permanent. In all cases, chemo brain is not a joke, but a challenging, long-term reality for many cancer patients receiving chemotherapy.

Chemo Class Acts

For years Wendy had undergone cancer treatments in California, from chemotherapy to bone-marrow transplant(s). She and her friends—chemo-buddies—had been through it all together! Today, Wendy was learning about a promising new treatment, and her friends had something special planned.

A limousine arrived at the medical center. Inside, Wendy's friends had lunch waiting as they whisked her off to Hollywood for a day at *The Price Is Right* studios. Special arrangements were made—no waiting in line and front row seats. Truly a chemo class act!

Here are some ways to create your own chemo class acts:

1. Leave a surprise gift for your survivor-friend at the chemo desk.
2. Deliver a decorative jar filled with lemon drops or hard candy to ward off nausea.
3. Make a date to bring a light lunch to the chemo center to enjoy together.
4. Give patients experiencing hair loss a sun hat with built-in UV sun ray protection.
5. Send long, beautiful head scarves to wear alone or wear over a knit cap.
6. Rummage through hospital and cancer center gift shops for everything from small, inspirational books to classy wigs and hats, from cancer cookbooks to comfortable post-surgery clothing!
7. Go wig shopping together. Try on colors or styles that are new, funky, and fun.

—B.

RADIATION THERAPY

Several years ago I was invited to speak to an undergraduate cancer class at Indiana University (Bloomington). A few months later, I joined the class on a field trip to visit the state-of-the-art Indiana University Health Cancer Radiation Center. Our hosts that evening were Kevin Rush, the administrative director of the radiation oncology center, and Jeffrey Mumper, the staff physicist.

I was astonished to watch Mr. Mumper create computer models—virtual patients—to determine how to deliver radiation most efficiently to tumors and avoid normal tissue. While touring this facility, I was also amazed by the technologic complexity and staff expertise required for today's radiation therapy treatments. After the tour, I asked Mr. Rush and Mr. Mumper if they would provide us with simple, straightforward answers to friends' questions about this complex field and the radiation therapy experience.

What Friends Want to Know

*by Kevin Rush, MHA, RT(R)(T), FASRT, and
Jeffrey Mumper, MS*

What is radiation and how is it used in cancer therapy?
Radiation is basically energy. In cancer therapy, the task is to kill the cancer (or prevent the cells' growth or reproduction) by bringing the radiation into a *specific* intersection point in the body where the tumor is located. Your friend's radiation team may be composed of a radiation oncologist, oncology nurse, radiation therapist, dosimetrist,[3] and physicist. In some cases, dietary counseling and massage therapy are also included. Radiation therapy can be used alone or in conjunction with chemotherapy and/or

---

[3] A dosimetrist calculates the proper dosage of radiation.

surgery, and over one-half to three quarters of cancer patients will undergo radiation therapy.[4]

Is there more than one type of radiation therapy?

Yes! Most radiation therapy patients are treated using external beam therapy from a linear accelerator that produces photon and electron radiation.

Some cancers in the brain and other locations are now being treated with highly focused radiation therapy using protons delivered by a cyclotron. Proton therapy avoids damaging sensitive nearby tissues.

What about the use of radioactive "seeds?"

Radioactive seeds are sometimes used for treating *prostate cancer*. They are implanted directly into the prostate. The radiation seeds remain in the patient but decay over time. Patients are asked to avoid close proximity to small children and pregnant women while the radiation decays, typically one to two days, at most.

Other patients may be treated using High Dose Rate brachytherapy (HDR). This type of therapy, using radioactive sources, is sometimes used for *gynecological cancers*. During treatment, your friend will have to remain in an isolated room with limited visitation times. In HDR treatment, however, the radioactive seed remains in the patient for the duration of the treatment only. The radiation does *not* remain with the patient when he or she returns home.

What side effects might my friend experience? Will he or she need to stay away from other people because of radioactivity?

Patients may have a reddening or drying out of the skin at the radiation site(s) or even slough off wet skin. Patients with head and neck cancer may experience dry mouth, thrush, mucus development, or even permanent dry mouth. Two to three hours after treatment,

---

[4] The National Cancer Institute reported, "Of the estimated 1.47 million Americans who will be diagnosed with cancer in 2009, 60–75 percent will undergo radiation therapy for their disease." *The NCI Cancer Bulletin* (September 8, 2009, Vol.6, No.7). http://www.cancer.gov.aboutnci/ncicancerbculletin/archive 2009/090809/page 8. Accessed 4/02/12.

patients often experience some fatigue. As treatments progress, patients are going to feel increasingly fatigued; they may feel great on Monday, but find they are dragging by Friday.

With the exception of patients with implanted radiation seeds, patients don't need to stay away from people, nor should they do so. (*See* the cautions listed previously in "What about the use of radioactive seeds?")

What happens during my friend's first visit to the radiation center?

Following consultation with a radiation oncologist, your friend will undergo a CT scan. He or she will return home while information from the scan goes into a computer. The computer then constructs a *virtual patient* to determine how to use the radiation to treat the cancer and avoid surrounding normal tissue. Once the plan is reviewed and approved by the radiation oncologist and checked by the radiation team, your friend will be ready to start treatment.

How often might my friend need radiation and how long will each treatment take?

Radiation treatments generally require patients to come in every day, Monday through Friday. Appointments usually last only fifteen minutes. The first treatment is longer because the radiation team will verify that the plan approved by the radiation oncologist can be delivered accurately by the treatment machine. Marks will also be placed on the patient that will be used for each day's treatment alignment.

During treatment your friend must stay in one position, usually for fifteen minutes each day. Immobilization devices will make your friend as comfortable as possible while keeping him or her stationary. The complete course of treatment may take as little as one day or as long as six to seven weeks. Once the full course of treatment is completed, some patients will have follow-up checks for up to five years.

A View from the Inside Out

by Julie Meek, PhD, RN, CNS

As a nursing educator I am well acquainted with cancer therapy treatments. I acquired a brand new perspective, however, when I became the patient undergoing radiation therapy. Below are seven tips for you to consider as we take a look at radiation therapy from the inside out.

Tip #1: The effects of radiation sometimes last as long as eighteen months; friends must recognize that the experience isn't *really* over when radiation treatments conclude.

Tip #2: The Hassle Factor. Many patients need to receive radiation treatments every day, five days a week, and depending upon the distance between a patient's home and the treatment center, travel can involve up to two to three hours a day. Furthermore, patients may need assistance in determining how to adjust work and family responsibilities so they fit into the radiation schedule.

Tip #3: Some patients may travel great distances for treatment, requiring them to stay in an apartment or hotel room near the treatment center, returning home only on weekends. In this instance, patients will have some down time to fill. Consider offering to travel with your patient-friend or to research information on things to do in the city of treatment. You may need to help your patient-friend explore housing options or secure financial assistance for travel and housing.

Tip #4: Patients undergoing radiation should know that they can choose their *marking method*—the way to delineate the area to receive radiation. Often tattoos are suggested, but if the person doesn't want this permanent reminder of the radiation experience, markings can be protected in other ways.

Tip #5: Help your patient-friend buy comfortable clothing for the area being radiated and do it early in the process. Encourage your friend to spend as little money as possible on this clothing, since the marking pens will permanently stain the clothing.

Tip #6: Encourage your patient-friend to do *all* the recommended skin care. Often the skin-care routine includes gentle washing and application of special creams three times a day. It's important to do this to protect against skin breakdown *later* in the radiation process.

Tip #7: Radiation oncologists need to understand how their patients are responding to treatment, including side effects, so encourage your patient-friend to keep a daily journal tracking symptoms, etc., in preparation for his next doctor visit.

Side Effects

Often it is not the cancer treatment itself, but the resulting side effects that most significantly impact normal day-to-day living for cancer patients. The National Cancer Institute lists over fifteen potential side effects for chemotherapy and half that many resulting from radiation treatments. What should friends know?

1. Side effects vary from patient to patient and occur in differing intensities. While one patient may suffer debilitating diarrhea, another will experience frustrating bouts of constipation.

2. While nausea was once a central part of the chemotherapy experience, today there are a host of anti-nausea drugs available. These drugs serve to reduce or alleviate nausea and vomiting during the course of chemotherapy.

3. Not every chemotherapy patient will lose his or her hair, either completely or partially. This side effect is directly related to the type and intensity of certain chemotherapy drugs. Radiation patients will only

lose hair found at the irradiated site unless they are receiving radiation to the head. In this case, they may lose their entire head of hair.

4. Dry mouth and mouth sores are common and patients are encouraged to rinse their mouths with salt-water and baking soda solutions several times a day to help alleviate mouth sores.

5. Chemotherapy often impacts patients' immune systems, making them prone to other illnesses or infections. Few people undergoing chemotherapy realize they should be careful around recently vaccinated young children. How long patients should avoid such contact depends upon the chemotherapy drugs they are receiving. Be certain to tell patient-friends to *check with their physicians* if they will be in contact with children or other people receiving live vaccines.

6. Chemotherapy patients may experience discoloration and even fungal or bacterial infections in fingernails and toenails.

7. Radiation patients may experience skin changes and are asked to keep treated areas covered whenever going outdoors. Both chemotherapy and radiation can make skin extra sensitive to sun exposure and sunscreen is a must. Loose clothing is also recommended. Skin changes may include redness, swelling, tenderness, or even blistering.

8. Chemo brain. Chemotherapy patients report varying degrees of memory loss, difficulties with motor skills, word recall, multi-tasking, and changes in the speed of cognitive processing. These symptoms occur both during treatment and afterwards.

9. Occasionally, chemotherapy patients will experience some neurological side effects. One such effect is peripheral neuropathy, a nerve condition. It is the result of damage to the small nerves which serve the

hands and feet. Most commonly it causes numbness and tingling and can cause difficulty with fine motor skills such as buttoning a shirt, turning pages, or typing. When severe, it can also affect patients' balance when walking. The neuropathy is often reversible after the chemotherapy is completed, but it can take months to sometimes a year or two to improve, and sometimes the damage can be permanent.

10. Appetites are easily affected by cancer treatments. Some patients will find eating difficult while others find themselves perpetually snacking. Who ever imagined they would gain weight during cancer treatments? It is common, right along with weight loss. Some patients also complain that foods taste different or that they find certain smells difficult to tolerate.

11. The most common side effect of treatment therapies is fatigue. For radiation therapy patients, fatigue increases as patients receive additional treatments. The effects of radiation treatments are often delayed so that patients may feel fine for the first couple of weeks of treatment and may not experience side effects until the end of the course of therapy. The side effects often continue to worsen for several weeks before they improve. The fatigue for radiation usually does not reach its maximum until two to four weeks *after* the treatment is completed.

12. Over time, chemotherapy patients may notice a somewhat predictable cycle for their side effects. In between treatments there may be times when side effects are most severe and times of relative freedom from these effects. Unfortunately, this is not true for all patients.

—B.

---

* General information for this sidebar was obtained from National Cancer Institute's website locations: http://www.cancer.gov/cancertopics/coping/chemo-side-effects and http://www.cancer.gov/cancertopics/coping/radiation-side-effects, (accessed February 17, 2012). Additional information was provided by Julie Monroe, MD, in written communication with the author, April 2, 2012.

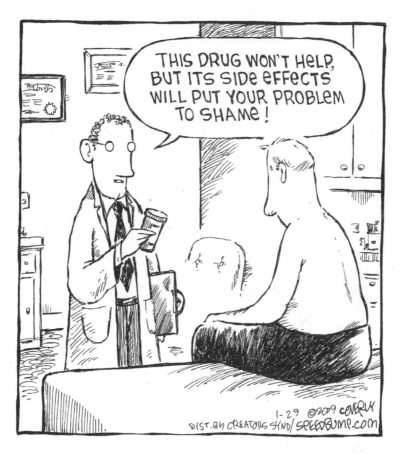

COMPLEMENTARY INTEGRATIVE MEDICINE

Although cancer treatment utilizes the expertise of specialists, cancer care practitioners are increasingly looking at the whole person. This has led to a new medical discipline called complementary integrative medicine.

Michael Finkelstein, MD, has a thoughtful and insightful approach to treating the whole patient. I visited him at Sun-Raven, the holistic health center he founded in Bedford, New York. There Dr. Finkelstein addressed both my questions about complementary integrative medicine and my concerns about non-traditional therapies.

What Friends Want to Know

by Michael Finkelstein, MD

What is complementary integrative medicine and why is it used in conjunction with traditional cancer therapies?
Integrative Medicine is an emerging discipline of medicine that is "healing-oriented, taking account of the whole person (body, mind, and spirit), including all aspects of lifestyle. It . . . makes use of all appropriate therapies, both conventional and alternative."[5]

Across the country, hospitals and cancer care centers are increasingly adopting complementary integrative approaches to treat cancer, reduce treatment side effects, manage pain, and improve overall health. Your friend's physician or cancer center may suggest or routinely offer one or more complementary therapies *in addition to* a planned standard course of treatment. Since these therapies are offered in conjunction with traditional therapies, such as chemotherapy or radiation, they are appropriately termed complementary integrative.

What are some common complementary integrative approaches?
Complementary approaches include energy work (reiki, therapeutic touch); acupuncture, acupressure, and reflexology; mind-body work (hypnotherapy, guided imagery, meditation, biofeedback); aromatherapy; supplements; and integrative movement (yoga, tai-chi, and qi gong), to name only a few.

Are all approaches safe, and what are some red flags of concern?
Friends need to be aware that alongside sound complementary integrative medical practices, *there are also practitioners or approaches that may be harmful.* Distinguishing credible practices from those

---

[5] V. Maizes and R.Horwitz, "Ethics, education and integrative medicine." 7 March 2006. Ethics JAMA. 2004; 6(11) http://www.ama-assn.org/ama/pub/category/13194.html

that are unreliable and/or misleading is important. Red flags of caution and concern should be raised whenever a patient chooses to stop a medically recommended cancer protocol *in favor of* an alternative approach or *when his or her choices are made out of desperation rather than knowledge*. While the autonomy of each individual should be respected, it is advisable to challenge such decisions (1) in either of the above situations, (2) when the alternative approaches are particularly costly, or (3) when there are *claims of cure*.

Twig Tea

It was Christmas, and Marilyn and her friends were arriving at the church for our weekly meeting. Each of us carried a small gift to exchange and something delicious to share. There were brownies, cookies, and other Christmas delights. Marilyn held a small bundle she was keeping warm in a swath of towels. We couldn't wait to see what it was.

"What did you bring, Marilyn?" I asked, as she unwrapped her "delight."

"Twig tea," she replied.

We all chimed in together, "*Twig* tea?"

"It's part of my macrobiotic diet. Try some. You'll like it." She set the pot down alongside the plates laden with sugary treats.

Well, we all tried some of the special tea, and it was okay, but twig tea certainly couldn't hold a candle to brownies, almond crescents, or even our standard cup of Earl Grey.

Over the coming months, our group consumed several more pots of twig tea, in support of Marilyn. But along with the tea came questions. What were these special diets and unusual treatment approaches Marilyn was embracing as she became more desperate for a cure? Karen, the nurse in our group, worried how her diet might be affecting Marilyn's overall health. Marilyn confided in us that she stashed chocolate bars around the house to snack on when she just couldn't take the rigid dietary restrictions anymore.

Marilyn embraced the world of complementary integrative medicine along with her standard cancer therapies; she also occasionally veered perilously close to the world of unregulated alternative medicine. We worried that she could fall prey to an alternative procedure or medication that would, in fact, deprive her of the help she actually needed.

In the end, Marilyn tried numerous complementary approaches while continuing with her standard therapies, but her cancer was simply too advanced. In her quest, however, she became our teacher. She taught us not to summarily dismiss practices we didn't understand (such as reiki, therapeutic touch, visualization, or even twig tea). And she also taught us not to hesitate to question and to research any approach that made us uncomfortable, particularly if it suggested it was a "cure" or substitute for standard cancer therapies. We learned there are many charlatans out there, but also there are some safe complementary approaches that helped Marilyn to lessen her pain and better handle treatment side effects.

It is a slippery slope we friends traverse. In the end, we have a dual responsibility: to support our patient-friends in their journey, while also helping them to recognize the dangers hidden in treatments that profess "cures," or require patients to suspend or stop standard cancer therapies and/or disregard physicians' counsel.

—B.

What are some considerations in evaluating non-traditional treatments?

Here are some questions that may help guide your friend in evaluating his or her options, particularly as they pertain to nonconventional approaches. Ask:

- How did you learn of this approach?
- What attracts you to this particular treatment or approach?
- What credentials and recommendations did you evaluate before selecting this practitioner?
- How open is the practitioner to discussing the approach with your medical doctor(s)?
- What are the risks accompanying this treatment?
- Does the proponent of this treatment have studies to back up claims of cures or treatment successes? Will you have direct access to former patients for references?
- Will the treatment, travel, or accompanying residence away from home put you or your family at personal or financial risk?
- How do you plan to integrate the approach with your current medical treatment?

During cancer treatment, it is important that an individual and his or her support team keep the process whole, considering the mind and spirit as well as the body. Ideally integrated with standard therapies, complementary integrative practices may hold important keys to a more positive and comfortable cancer experience for your friend.

The Cleveland Clinic Cancer Center, in conjunction with cancer survivor Scott Hamilton, provides an easily understood explanation of complementary medicine on the website www.chemocare.com/complementarymedicine.asp. The National Cancer Institute also offers general information and questions to consider at: www.cancer.gov. (Type CAM in the search box).

The Best Treatment Possible

Several years ago, I interviewed a Montana farmer in his late sixties. Bob was a colon cancer survivor. When diagnosed, he had made a decision to seek the best treatment he could find and afford—even if it meant leaving his small rural community. Bob and his wife decided to travel east to Rochester, Minnesota, for his treatment. Years later, they remained firmly convinced that this decision was responsible for Bob's survival.

Bob told me, "In small rural communities, physicians may be unaware of—or reluctant to embrace—newer technologies and treatments. They may be hesitant to refer patients to larger, out-of-town hospitals or cancer centers. It is often up to the patients themselves to request a second opinion and to explore additional treatment options and/or treatment facilities."

Fortunately, Bob's physician was upfront and honest with him. "You may want to go to Mayo," he said. "Somebody there may be able to figure this out, but I can't."

Bob agreed, and he and his wife, Barbara, headed to Rochester, even though it meant leaving home for an extended period of time. While Bob received treatment at the Mayo Clinic, he and Barbara settled into temporary housing. Their neighbors regularly sent them videos of the farm (including taped interviews with the kids) just to assure them everything was okay.

When treatment finally concluded, Bob and Barbara said good-bye to their health care team. They boarded the train for the 900 mile trip back from Minneapolis to Montana. When they finally arrived the next afternoon, they were tired, but delighted to be back.

As they stepped off the train, they couldn't believe their eyes. The platform was crowded with townspeople. The whole town—kids and grownups—had come to the station to welcome Bob and Barbara home.

While this story is set in rural America, its message is important for all cancer patients. It reminds us of two things:

1. **Patient-friends should routinely ask for a second opinion.** Most physicians support this approach. When asked, many doctors will help their patients

find a cancer specialist who will review test results and offer a second opinion without delay.

2. **Everyone facing cancer should receive the best treatment he or she can access and afford.** It is ultimately the *patient's* decision as to which treatment to pursue, and whether a local or regional facility would be best. Friends, however, may volunteer to gather information on local and regional cancer facilities, clinical trials, and treatment options. In this way, you help keep patients fully informed, enabling them to be certain *their* decisions are also *sound* decisions.

—B.

PART FOUR

WHEN LIFE DRAWS
TO A CLOSE

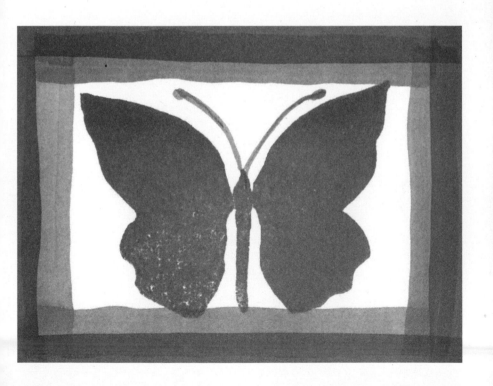

Chapter Eight

PREPARING FOR THE END OF LIFE AND THE GIFT OF PEACE

LETTING GO, GRIEVING, AND PHASES OF DYING

When a friend's cancer is deemed terminal, we experience many emotions over the impending loss—sadness, anger, disbelief. A diagnosis of terminal cancer, however, doesn't necessarily mean your friend will die this week, this month, or even this year. What happens first is that you, and everyone else who cares for your friend, will begin the long and agonizing process of letting go—giving up long-held dreams and expectations that are part of the tapestry of friendship. Anticipating the loss of a friend's love, comfort, and companionship sets in motion the twin processes of letting go and of grieving.

Rev. David Jenkins, retired head of M.D. Anderson Cancer Center's chaplaincy department (Houston, Texas), says, "The terminal phase of cancer is not so much the management of a dreadful disease, though that is important, as it is the complex process of letting go, which includes grieving, mixed with gratitude for the gift of life."[1]

At the beginning of this chapter you will learn what to expect when a friend's life draws to a close, appropriate ways to respond, and what it means to grieve. You will also find information on hospice and ways to promote a sense of peace during cancer and at the end of life.

I traveled to a premier hospice network located in Phoenix, Arizona—Hospice of the Valley. There I met Meredith Rivers,[2] who introduced me to grief counselors Marty Tousley and Rev. Steven Averill. In our conversations and subsequent correspondence, they shared their expertise and that of others in the Hospice of the Valley network, to help us understand phases of dying and the important process of grieving.

Journeying toward the End of Life

Hospice of the Valley[3]

The actual physical process of dying often starts two weeks prior to death. Family and friends, however, may notice psychological or emotional changes in the preceding months. The patient may spend time reflecting on end-of-life issues and on his or her beliefs regarding what happens next. You may notice your patient-friend withdrawing or beginning to separate from the world around him. At this time he or she may begin to sleep more as the body slows down and may spend most of the day in bed.

What can you do? When your friend is alert and awake, try to be there. Patients often find comfort and reassurance in having people

---

[1] Rev. David Jenkins in conversation with the author, Houston, Texas, 2006.

[2] Meredith Rivers is Director of Clinical Support Services, Hospice of the Valley, Phoenix, Arizona.

[3] With appreciation to Hospice of the Valley for permission to adapt material for this section from *Final Days: Sharing the Journey* (Phoenix, AZ: Hospice of the Valley, 2008). Used by permission.

nearby, even when they're just sitting quietly. *Touch* becomes more important than words. Hold hands. Play or sing music he or she enjoys.

Sometimes your friend may not want to eat or drink anything. (It also isn't unusual for a very ill person to ask for particular foods, only to refuse them when they arrive.) If your friend is confused about time, place, and the identity of people, don't be alarmed. Answer questions calmly. Say your name and describe what you are going to do before you do it.

One or two weeks prior to death, as patient-friends begin separating from the physical world, restlessness and confusion may set in. Again, this is a form of letting go. Your friend may pull at the bed linen, talk with loved ones who have died, or describe taking a symbolic trip "home." Much of the time, your friend will be asleep. Be present, open, and loving; offer reassurance.

As death approaches, the physical body undergoes changes. Hearing is the last of the five senses to be lost, so never say anything you would not want your friend to hear, even if he or she appears comatose. You may also notice that breathing is becoming irregular and there may be rattling sounds or coughing. This can be distressing for you to hear, but is not painful to the patient.

Some people experience a surge of energy within days or hours prior to death. Your friend may sit up, speak clearly, or eat a meal. Maintain an environment that your friend likes—TV on or off; silence or favorite music; photos of loved ones displayed on the walls; religious or spiritual symbols; and prayers or rituals that are meaningful. Touch, hold, and comfort one another. See this time as an opportunity to express important feelings to one another and to reaffirm all that your relationship has meant. Reassure your friend that he or she will be forever remembered, and remain forever close at heart.

A Gift of Love

My own father was hospitalized at eighty-eight years of age. Dad lived with chronic leukemia, heart disease, and bladder cancer for many years. He remained very active. He worked in the church office every Wednesday and served as treasurer for a local foundation up until his passing. With a keen mind and sharp memory, he rarely missed a beat, and we all knew that!

Once in the hospital, however, it took Dad a full week to convince our family that he was indeed dying, and that he was okay with that. We continued to encourage him to fight on, saying, "You can do it! We're here for you." Our family simply wasn't ready to face Dad's approaching death, and he knew this. We weren't ready to let go. So, he continued to prod us to become as realistic and accepting of the end of life, as he was. He spoke of experiences and dreams he was having in the hospital that nurtured his sense of awe and anticipation, rather than a fear of death. When Mom finally made the decision to place him in hospice care, he turned to her and said, "Thank You!" He was ready to say good-bye, and his family was now on board with that decision.

Sometimes the best support family and friends can provide for terminal cancer patients is to say the words, "It's okay to let go. We will miss you and we'll always love you, but we will be okay." This may be the very gift of love they have been waiting to receive.

—B.

LEARNING ABOUT GRIEF

A Conversation with Marty Tousley

Because we spend most of our lives denying the reality of death—and our culture reinforces this—most of us don't know how to grieve. However, we must learn how to do so in order to go on with our own lives after a friend passes.

No one is ever fully prepared for the death of a friend or a loved one. As your friend nears death—or when he or she passes away—you will experience a time of grieving. In *Grieving the Death of a Friend*, author Harold Ivan Smith says that "friendgrief" can be devastating.[4]

---

[4]   Harold Ivan Smith coins the word "friendgrief" in his book *Grieving the Death of a Friend* (Augsburg Fortress: Minneapolis. 1996).

You may feel angry, sad, lonely, confused and/or bewildered. You may find it hard to believe your friend is gone; you may even pick up the phone before you remember he or she is no longer there to take your call.

Grief is demanding work. As you begin to grieve, it is important to understand what you are experiencing. I asked bereavement counselor Marty Tousley to help us understand four common situations that may arise during your grieving process.[5]

Situation #1: I can't eat or sleep since my friend died. I keep wondering, "who's next?" How long will it be before I can move on with my life?

Ms. Tousley: Grief is extremely powerful. It can catch you totally unprepared, knock you off balance, and shake you to the core. It can affect you—physically, emotionally, socially, and spiritually. Grief serves to remind you how fragile life is and how vulnerable you are to loss. It can lead you to question the meaning of your own life.

Grief work is very hard and it takes enormous energy. You cannot wait it out; you won't get over it quickly, and nobody can do it for you. It is called grief work because finding your way through grief is hard work. The longer you wait, the harder it becomes. Be gentle with yourself as you grieve. Give yourself sufficient time and space to experience your loss as you gradually work through it.

Situation #2: My friends and I seem to be grieving very differently. Is there a proper way to grieve?

Ms. Tousley: Grief is a normal, yet highly personal response to loss. How grief is expressed varies among individuals. Everyone grieves differently depending on age, gender, personality, culture, value system, past experience with loss, and available support. Grieving differs even among members of the same family. It is a natural process, and depending on how it is managed and understood, it can lead to healing and personal growth.

---

[5]   Used by permission. Based upon the book, *Finding Your Way Through Grief,* 2nd edition, © 2008 by Marty Tousley Ms. Tousley is a bereavement counselor with Hospice of the Valley, Phoenix, AZ and serves as moderator of its online grief discussion forums. Her bereavement website is: www.griefhealing.com.

Situation #3:   It has been two months since my friend, Judy, died. I still cry for her, and I talk about her a lot. Should I shut myself away until my grief has passed?

Ms. Tousley: Effective grieving is not done alone. Friends and family members may be finished with your grief long before you are finished with your need to talk about it. It is important that you find an understanding listener to whom you can express your feelings and experiences. If friends and family are not as available as you need them to be, or if your need exceeds their capacity to help, consider finding a counselor or a grief support group.

Situation #4:   My friend died but I still sense her presence from time to time. Is this unusual?

Ms. Tousley: Death may have ended your friend's life, but it did not end your relationship. The bond you and your friend have will continue and endure throughout your lifetime, as your shared memories and past experiences accompany you into the future. Many grievers report maintaining an active connection with their deceased loved ones by talking to them, dreaming about them, sensing their presence, or feeling watched over and protected by them.

Your pattern of progressing through your grief will be uneven, unpredictable, and unique, with no specific time frame. But the more you learn about grief, the better you can cope with it. When you understand what is happening to you, you will feel more in control of your grief and in a better position to take care of yourself.

Movements in the Healing Process

by Steven D. Averill, MDiv, FT

The first movement of the healing process is becoming aware of one's feelings and the reality of the loss. There is an initial numbing effect immediately following a loss, perhaps along with disbelief, denial, shock, and separation anxiety. However, once you can step back and observe the feelings that are flowing through you and see the reality of the loss, the healing process has begun. This awareness comes slowly as the layers of disbelief are sloughed off and you begin to realize that the pain of the loss is not unbearable (although waves of seemingly unbearable pain may still occur).

Telling the story of one's loss is integral to healing. *Acknowledging the pain*, instead of denying it, is what allows a person to move through it.

There is no denying that after losing a friend, you are confronted with finding a new way of living without that friend. You may even experience feelings of guilt when you no longer think of your friend every day. Allow yourself to see your loss in a greater context of meaning. Moving beyond your grief is an essential spiritual task in the process of healing.

In the web of life, we are all connected. Becoming involved in reaching out to others who are experiencing loss in their lives is the final movement in the healing process. While healing requires our taking responsibility for moving through our own pain, we also need others to complete the process. Receiving and giving support is the final step towards healing in the face of profound loss.

HOSPICE: WHAT FRIENDS SHOULD KNOW

by Benjamin Ranck, MD, and Rev. William Griffith, MDiv, DMin

A model hospice program is Hospice of South Central Indiana (Columbus). There I spoke with the program's retired medical director, Benjamin Ranck, MD, and chaplain Rev. William Griffith. I asked them to give us a thumb-nail sketch of what it means to be in hospice care and how friends can appropriately respond when visiting someone in hospice.

Hospice: Sandy's Story

When I first talked with Sandy, she had been struggling with recurring breast cancer for more than five years. We were having supper in a coffee shop near her home, and although she looked good, I could see the lines of worry worn into her face.

She looked directly into my eyes. "Bonnie, I want a miracle," she said. "I want to know why others have one. How do I get one? Where do I sign up?"

I shook my head. I had no answers to give to her.

Sandy had traveled from Indiana to Houston's M.D. Anderson Cancer Center and, after months of treatment, had exhausted all hopes of a cure. Now she was facing the realities of terminal cancer. She was experiencing a great sense of loss. She was also tired and a little scared.

We talked of many things, but finally got around to how she was coping with the realization that her own life was drawing to a close. Her shoulders slumped as she let out a sigh. "It's very tough having to make your death okay for others," she said. "You can't always share your real feelings . . . they can't deal with it."

We talked for over an hour and a half. As we prepared to part, Sandy said, "Thanks for listening and for letting me speak frankly."

"I have to go back East," I said, "but let's stay in touch." Sandy promised she would.

A few weeks later she emailed me: "I have gone now into the hospice program—Hard! Hard! More grieving. Having more fullness in my gut and some pain. I have been given meds for pain as needed. It's very difficult to succumb to everything."

In the very next sentence, however, I was surprised to read, "On the bright side, Pete, the kids, and I took a 5-day cruise . . . to St. John, New Brunswick, and Halifax, Nova Scotia."

While her experiences appeared inconsistent, even improbable, they pointed straight to the heart of hospice: Sandy's hospice care team was helping control her pain to make Sandy comfortable. In this way, she and her family could experience a good quality of life during her remaining weeks. For Sandy and her family, hospice was making all the difference.

—B.

What is hospice care?

Many people think hospice is a place where patients go to die. In truth, hospice is often not a *place* at all, but rather a comprehensive philosophy of care for the seriously ill. Hospice programs offer *palliative care,* that is, specialized care focusing on quality of life and comfort, rather than cure. The length of hospice care varies from days or weeks to periods as long as six months.[6]

Hospice is a unique interdisciplinary approach. It addresses total suffering—both physical and non-physical. Acting as a team, health care professionals work to meet the physical, social, psychological, and spiritual needs of patients. The team may include

---

[6]   Medicare generally provides hospice benefits to patients with six months or less to live assuming their disease runs its normal course. These benefits may be extended under certain circumstances. Certain in-patient hospice facilities have limits as to the length of time patients can remain at the facility, and therefore, patients may be released from the facilities to receive further care at home or in another care facility.

a physician-medical director, nurse, home health aide, social worker, and chaplain. A host of individualized services, treatments or medications, and support are available to make patients as pain-free and comfortable as possible. Additionally, the hospice team goes to where a patient is living, whether that is at home, in a community care facility, or a hospice in-patient facility. Each team member works with the patient and his or her family to identify the patient's needs.

When people accept their end of life diagnoses, they are able to plan for the best use of the time that remains. Hospice care was created to help seriously ill people live as fully as possible during their remaining lifetime. At the end of life, hospice care helps people die peacefully and with dignity.

How to Respond

One of the most important things we can do when a friend has an incurable illness is to listen effectively and to understand as much as we can about our friends' fears, hopes, and goals. We gain true compassion when we listen with understanding. Your questions should be shaped in a way that gives the patient permission to be honest when answering. Ask, "What have you been thinking about lately or during your quiet moments?" This gives your friend permission to share thoughts and feelings honestly. It also communicates your willingness to walk alongside your friend even when the going gets tough.

Hospice provides an empathetic atmosphere in which patients and family members are free to speak what is on their minds: to question, examine issues, explore solutions, laugh, cry, and voice their deepest concerns—without fear of rejection, isolation, or abandonment. As friends, we should also do our best to create a similar environment of acceptance and honesty.[7]

---

[7]   Hospice helps to set a stage for enhancing and strengthening sources of meaning. This is a time patients may want to engage in spiritual conversations or seek spiritual or religious rituals to help them celebrate their beliefs and values. Hospice also helps bring orderly closure to a patient's affairs, by aiding in the transfer of fiscal, legal, and social responsibilities and addressing family needs. After the death of their loved one, hospice also meets families' continuing bereavement needs.

The palliative care that hospice provides ensures that patients live their last days in the best way they can and that families have a sounding board and a broad shoulder for their grief.

Hospice as Holy Time

Death doesn't always come easily. Sometimes it roars and rips at your heart and soul. But when it comes softly on tip-toes and gently lifts up a dying patient, it can be a beautiful thing.

It was time to stop the *whrrrr* of the oxygen machine and to settle into the quiet. The decision had been made to stop treatment. Bill would be moving to hospice within the hour.

As if on cue, Pastor Susan approached the hospital room quietly and asked if she could see Bill. He seemed especially pleased to see her this one last time. They only spoke a few words, as Bill was conserving his energy. But it was enough.

Susan turned to Bill's wife and said, "You are entering a holy time." We don't think of hospice or even the end of life as "holy time," and yet somehow it fit perfectly. Life was drawing to a close, and with all the accompanying sadness, somehow there was a certain symmetry to it—a life well-lived was coming full circle.

Bill moved to the hospice facility that afternoon, and his wife and two grown children sat with him throughout the evening and on into the wee hours of the morning. The room was quiet and peaceful with soft lighting—a sharp contrast to the ICU's bright lights and incessant motion. The hospice staff was just down the hall—available, attentive, but never intrusive. Bill's nurse was respectful, speaking directly to Bill, always calling him by name when explaining what was happening or about to happen.

The hours moved slowly as the children took turns holding one of their father's hands, while their mother held the other. It was "holy time" as Susan had said, and it was precious. And then, just eight hours after entering hospice, Bill's lungs took in a final gentle breath, and he was gone. Just like that, in a holy moment. Through their tears his family expressed their gratitude—gratitude for a peaceful passing, gratitude for hospice, and gratitude for holy moments to treasure now and always.

—*B.*

THE GIFT OF PEACE

When life is drawing to a close, we desperately want to give friends the gift of abiding peace—peace of mind, body, and soul. The hard truth is that peace is not ours to give; we can only facilitate its coming. As a trusted friend, however, you can act as a vital catalyst, helping patient-friends develop their own emerging sense of peace. I asked chaplain Rev. David Jenkins to suggest several ways friends can help.[8] He mentioned three things:

1. Help patient-friends move toward an *acceptance of what is*. But first, it is important to recognize acceptance requires different things at different times in life. For patients starting on the cancer journey, acceptance may stem from knowing there are cutting-edge treatments and clinical trials available to them.[9] You can help research these options. Later in the cancer journey, you can encourage patient-friends' acceptance of "what is" by helping them complete *unfinished business*—from "bucket lists" to visiting former classmates, homes, or favorite haunts.

---

[8]   David Jenkins in conversation with the author, Houston, Texas, March, 2006. David Jenkins is the retired head of the chaplaincy department at M.D. Anderson Cancer Center.

[9]   See the appendix for listings of comprehensive cancer centers and websites for clinical trial information.

Friends and family did just that for Hazel, 87, and William, 88. These two planned a final trip back to the Midwest. Once there, they wanted their son-in-law to drive them to Milwaukee to complete a bucket-list item. They wanted to see the law firm still bearing Hazel's father's name.

Unbeknownst to the couple, a friend contacted the firm to give them a "heads up." The current staff pulled out all the stops: They filmed a 40-minute "historical" video interview with Hazel and they arranged a surprise reunion between Hazel and her father's protégé (now well into his nineties). To top it off, the staff shared with them an album of priceless photos of Hazel's parents in their prime. The couple then headed out to Hazel's former home, where the new owners welcomed them with open arms.

Afterwards, Hazel said this special trip brought her the sense of closure she had sought for years.

2. Encourage patients' *reconciliation with all that has been.* Reconciliation is requisite to peace in every phase of life. Mending fences and repairing relationships is especially critical at the end of life. When patient-friends voice a desire for a reunion or reconciliation, you can step forward to help.

It happened many years ago to a family torn apart by a troublesome child, Frank.

Frank had always been the family pariah, in trouble with the law, and on the outs with his extended family. Few family members could even tell you where he was living from year to year. One day, word came that Frank was dying in a hospital thousands of miles away in Albuquerque. His father refused to go and see him, but his mother felt a tug on her heart that only a mother can know. She knew this reconciliation was important not only for Frank, but for herself as well. In her late seventies and traveling alone for the first time, she boarded a plane headed for Albuquerque and went to visit him.

There she met Frank's second wife, who spoke of how her son had transformed his life in the past few years. Frank had become a caring husband and he brought her a rose every night. They had a wonderful, loving relationship. While other family members remained skeptical, Frank's mother knew the time for recriminations was past. This was a unique opportunity to heal a relationship between a mother and a wayward son before it was too late.

When Frank's mother returned from Albuquerque, the family was amazed to see the degree of peace the trip had brought her.

3. Nurture patients' *confidence to face whatever will be.* Again, this element takes shape in varying ways. For patients with children, confidence in the future often rests in the certainty that their children will continue to have the love and care they require, no matter what their parent's prognosis. It may come from knowing dear friends will act as surrogates for them—helping a daughter prepare for her wedding or standing-in to witness a son's graduation. It can include entrusting friends with special letters or gifts intended to be opened on birthdays or other life milestones, even after the parent has passed.

For older patients, confidence in the future comes with the knowledge that their partners' or aging spouses' complex medical or personal needs will continue to be met. For still others, confidence in the future resides firmly in the long-held promises and practices inherent in patients' faith traditions (such as the Christian belief in life-after-death). Although some requests or beliefs may seem foreign to us, we foster final peace by honoring and respecting patients' deeply held beliefs and end-of-life requests, as best we can.

GIFTS OF PEACE DURING THE JOURNEY

Although we can't guarantee lasting peace in the midst of cancer's chaos, we can provide peaceful interludes and much needed respites for patients and their families during the journey. Recently, I was privileged to share one such interlude with my dear friend and editor, Rachel.

In December, Rachel was diagnosed with pancreatic cancer. As both a survivor and friend, I soon decided it was time for a visit. For two and a half months, Rachel had been experiencing a roller coaster ride of undulating emotions, difficult diagnoses, and brutal chemotherapy side effects. It was time for me to take a long weekend and fly to Manhattan to help share some peace and joy with Rachel.

While there, I visited her every day and we laughed for hours on end about the indignities of cancer: diets that more closely resemble baby food than adult fare and bathroom vanities where Chanel No. 5 is shoved aside to make room for practical comforts. We also spent time sitting quietly side-by-side, soaking up the late afternoon sun as it streamed through the apartment windows. And we talked about our families, our work, and our dreams.

Our three days together seemed like a week's vacation for both of us. When I returned home, Rachel said this time spent together had helped her to turn a corner. She was now energized to move on to face whatever might lie ahead.

More than anything, I wanted to assure Rachel that everything would be okay, but I couldn't. I could only provide daily respites filled with love, friendship, and laughter. As Rachel's health continued to decline over the next few months, we were increasingly grateful for this time together and our memories of that peaceful interlude.

Although you may not have the time or resources to fly across the country, there are many other ways to encourage a sense of peace during cancer. Here are eight taken from focus groups and friends' experiences:

Peaceful Environment As Marilyn's strength declined, she spent increasing amounts of time resting on the living room sofa. She wanted to surround herself with a soothing environment. With a little help from friends, she created a peaceful space by placing a small bamboo plant and a tiny tabletop fountain on the coffee table adjacent to the sofa. The sounds of softly cascading water amid bright greens shoots brought peace not only to Marilyn, but to her visitors as well.

Hope and Peace Nooy was struggling with late-stage colon cancer. Every Wednesday her husband, Michael, sent an email inviting over one-hundred friends to "Thursday Night with Nooy." After an update on her condition, Mike concluded these weekly emails with, "Tomorrow is Thursday and I hope that you can join us between 8:00 and 8:30 PM Eastern Time, to send Nooy as much good energy, and as many blessings as possible."

Nooy and Michael spent this half-hour each Thursday, in meditation and prayer at their home in Boston, knowing others were thinking of them. Repeatedly Michael wrote of the strong sense of peace and the immense comfort they experienced during these times of shared caring. After Nooy's passing, Nooy's family continued to draw strength from the love and concern demonstrated during a winter and spring filled with "Thursday Nights with Nooy."

Sounds of Peace Gladys was in a coma. The nursing staff called her family and asked for any suggestions as to how they might "reach her" or provide her with some comfort and solace. A former classical pianist, Gladys loved music all her life. "Try some classical music," her granddaughter said. That evening the staff turned on a soothing, classical CD. They reported it was only then that Gladys visibly relaxed and even responded slightly to those around her.

Bucket-List Trip Ernestine was in her nineties and her final wish was to ride around the old neighborhood in style. She asked a younger friend, Renee, to escort her on a special day out. So one sunny California afternoon, they climbed into Renee's shiny Pontiac two-seater, put the top down, and turned the music up. Renee said, "We were quite the sight: two sassy black ladies on the ride of a lifetime!"

A Peaceful Spin Lorraine was confined to a wheelchair. Like Ernestine, she wanted to tour her neighborhood one last time. So friends bundled Lorraine up, and together they took her out on a final "spin" around the block, wheelchair and all.

More Hope and Peace Kim, an elderly Korean woman, was terminally ill with cancer. The pastor asked her congregation to write personal notes to Kim; they also collected photographs, poems, and quotations of peace and hope. They placed these items in a lovely album entitled "Hope and Peace." The congregation presented it to the family as a reminder of the love surrounding them.

A Drawer Full of Hope and Peace Betty's partner, Joan, is struggling with a debilitating cancer. Over the years Joan has received hundreds of cards and well-wishes. She keeps them all in a huge drawer in her living room coffee table. Whenever Joan feels "down," she opens the drawer and rereads the cards and notes, renewing her hope and peace every time.

Symbolic Peace Japanese folklore suggests that a thousand folded paper cranes will summon good health. While being treated for cancer, Bonnie's overseas friends folded and sent colorful origami peace cranes. She displayed the cranes, enjoying their beauty and hope-filled prophesy. After her recovery, she gave the cranes to others experiencing cancer.

Whether you prepare an album, take a friend out for a drive, or pause each Thursday evening to remember a patient-friend in thought or prayer, you are facilitating a sense of peace and sharing an immeasurable gift of friendship when it is most needed.

TRUE REFUGE:
SEEKING PEACE WITH REV. SUSAN JI-ON POSTAL

Stress accompanies every phase of the cancer journey. No one is immune—not patients, their families, or friends. I wanted to know how to find peace in the midst of the stresses of cancer, so I traveled to the Empty Hand Zen Center in New Rochelle, New York. Housed in a small two-story brick building on a little side street, the center is surrounded by a lovely garden. It is an oasis of tranquility in the middle of a busy, urban area.

I walked up the path and I knocked on the door. A Zen Buddhist priest appeared. She was wearing a dark flowing robe and her hair was closely cropped. She was the essence of peace and serenity.

"Welcome," she said. "I am Rev. Susan Ji-on Postal, the center's teacher-in-residence."

Rev. Postal invited me into a large room. The space was simple but elegant with polished floors and rows of cushions and chairs for meditation. As the door closed behind us, the sounds of the city disappeared, replaced by total and complete silence. I took a seat across from Rev. Postal. I was told she suffered from a debilitating chronic illness so I asked her, "How we can find peace in the midst of serious illness?"

Rev. Postal took a moment to enter stillness, and then began to speak.

"One of Buddha's fundamental teachings is of 'Two Truths,' she said. "These twin truths infuse all of life:

"(1)   the Relative (you and I, good and bad, birth and death)
"(2)   the Ultimate, (no-separation, of One-body).

"Most of the time, we are caught in the relative level—caught up in *our* thinking, *our* stories, *our* fears. Meditation helps us to move beyond this. Living with the difficulty of illness, we have the opportunity to really see that who we are is not just *our thoughts* and *our story*. We have the opportunity to experience a bigger picture."

"How do we do this?" I asked.

"Becoming fully aware and *present in the moment*, practicing meditation and the *mindfulness of breathing* are first steps," she replied. "Through these practices, we can begin to take rest, to take true refuge in the boundlessness and peacefulness always available in every moment."

We talked a while longer and then took a walk in the garden. After I left, I began to recognize the importance of meditation during cancer. I sought out books by the Vietnamese Zen Master, Thich Nhat Hanh, books that provide simple examples of meditations for beginners (e.g., *The Miracle of Mindfulness*).

I also explored several other wonderful meditative practices— yoga, sign chi do, and tai chi. All are valuable, but no matter which meditative discipline you choose, the lesson remains the same. When you are in the midst of cancer's chaos, *take a moment to take a breath*. It will start you on a new path toward experiencing the peace that can be found in every moment—even during cancer.

Chapter Nine

THE GIFT OF REMEMBRANCE

REMEMBRANCE

Yizkor (Memorial) Service

In the rising of the sun and its going down, we remember them.

In the blowing of the wind and the chill of winter, we remember them.

In the opening of buds and in the rebirth of spring, we remember them.

In the blueness of the sky and in the warmth of summer, we remember them.

In the rustling of the leaves and in the beauty of autumn, we remember them.

In the beginning of the year and when it ends, we remember them.

When we are weary and in need of strength, we remember them.

When we are lost and sick at heart, we remember them.

When we have joys we yearn to share, we remember them.

So long as we live they too shall live, for they are now a part of us, as we remember them.[1]

As life draws to a close, patients often find comfort and reassurance in remembering—calling to mind valued relationships, the things that made life worthwhile, the accomplishments of which they are most proud, and even childhood memories. And when a patient dies, remembrance and ritual become a critical part of the grieving process for family and friends left behind.

A Tuscarora Indian proverb declares, "They are not dead who live in the hearts they leave behind."[2] How do you create these special times to remember your loved ones? I spoke with Elaine Amerson, EdD,[3] who has studied the importance of rituals in everyday living and in grieving. We discussed why it is important to have occasions to remember.

Dr. Amerson says, "We all realize that we have transforming rites of passage in our lives, such as our first job, a child's marriage, or a grandchild's graduation. These are the markers by which we measure our lives, and they are often accompanied by meaningful

---

[1] "In the rising of the sun" by Rabbi Sylvan Kamens and Rabbi Jack Riemer from *Gates of Repentence: The New Union Prayerbook* for the Days of Awe © 1978, 1996 by the Central Conference of American Rabbis is under the copyright protection of the Central Conference of American Rabbis and reprinted for use by permission of the CCAR. All rights reserved.

[2] Guy Zona, *The Soul Would Have No Rainbow if the Eyes Had No Tears and Other Native American Proverbs* (New York: Simon and Schuster, 1994), 23.

[3] Elaine Amerson, EdD, is a national education consultant, living and working in the Chicago area.

practices that provide opportunities to express our joy and to celebrate. However, sometimes we need specific rituals to express our
sorrow and mourning.

"When friends pass away, we add honor and reverence to
their memories through rituals of remembrance—opportunities
to celebrate and commemorate lives and relationships we never
want to forget. For centuries, final good-byes and mourning have
been marked by rituals, such as sitting shivah,[4] attending funerals,
visiting those in mourning, and participating in memorial services.
These practices provide meaningful times of grieving, comfort,
healing, and remembrance, all in the company of friends and
family."

Putting Dr. Amerson's advice into practice this past winter,
I helped organize a special service of remembrance and day of
events to honor Bill. Bill and his wife, Hazel, were in their late
eighties and had survived cancer numerous times: two bouts of
breast cancer for Hazel, bladder cancer and chronic leukemia for
Bill. They had been married sixty-six years when Bill passed away,
a few days before Christmas.

It was the day of Bill's memorial service, and Hazel just wanted
to get through it. Hazel and Bill's children had worked hard to
make this day a special one of remembrance, peace, and closure
for their mother. We decorated the chapel with tall turquoise and
sand-colored pillar candles—one for Bill, one for Hazel, and three
more representing their children. Interspersed among the tall
candles were eight half pillars, one for each of their grandchildren, and a small votive for each great-grandchild. The result was
beautiful and soothing and spoke clearly of "family."

I remember when Hazel stepped into the chapel, steeling herself for the hardest day of her life. She took a seat in the front row
between her children as the service began. The candles were lit,
beautiful music resounded, and words of remembrance, gratitude,
and hope were spoken. It was a moving and uplifting memorial.

---

[4] Shivah is a Jewish ritual of mourning in which the bereaved family remains at home for
the first days following burial of a close family member. During this time friends and
neighbors sit and visit with them in their grief.

When it concluded, fifty or so attendees stepped out into a glorious Arizona afternoon and travelled to a nearby restaurant. There they gathered in small groups, many around a "remembrance table" filled with fifty framed photographs of Bill and his family throughout the years. One of Bill's daughter's had scattered additional candid photos on individual dining tables to stimulate more memories.

Hazel sat down as her friends brought her a plate of hors d'oeuvres, sandwiches, and a welcome martini. For the next two hours, the dining room echoed with humorous anecdotes, stories of Bill, lots of hugs, and occasional tears.

After lunch, a number of guests went out to play a round of golf in Bill's honor. (It was Bill's favorite sport.) An impromptu barbeque was planned at a second daughter's home for later in the day. When Hazel arrived late in the afternoon, the patio was already filled with the laughter of children, grandchildren, and cousins—everyone reminiscing. The afternoon and evening were relaxed and fun-filled, and it was nine-thirty before Hazel was ready to go home.

At the door, Hazel turned to her daughter. Her eyes were rimmed with tears.

"Thank you," she said. "This could have been the worst day of my life, and instead it was one of the best."

Her daughter smiled and hugged her mother. Together, family and friends had accomplished all had they set out to do—to create places where Hazel could both remember and grieve, supported by loving friends and family.

Like Bill's golf tournament, the family barbeque, and the tables filled with photographs, friends and families are finding creative ways to remember loved ones while honoring their special interests, their accomplishments, and their faith. Here are a few more examples:

Favorite Color Eight-year-old Cameron struggled with cancer for much of his young life. His Virginia community held fundraising events to help his family, and when Cameron died, friends wondered how to support his family in their grief. A beautiful memorial service was planned, and attendees were asked to wear blue, Cameron's favorite color. At the service the family was enveloped in a sea of blue, tangible evidence of the community's continuing love and support.

Town Hall Remembrance Sandy was deeply attracted to many artistic mediums—from photography to fine art to textiles. Throughout her cancer experience, she used her artistic gifts as an outlet for her pain and grief. She also used her art to help others understand what it means to have cancer.

After her passing Sandy's family rented the town hall in their small New Hampshire community. There they created an exhibit of Sandy's collages, masks, paintings, and photographs—many inspired by her cancer journey. The family invited their community to join them in remembering Sandy, her life, and her work. It was a wonderful event. It served both as window to the cancer experience, and as a testimony to Sandy's resolve *never* to let cancer stifle her spirit.

Ohio Community Remembrance Linda was a highly respected attorney and public education advocate in Akron, Ohio. In lieu of a church funeral, her family invited the community to gather at the high school auditorium to memorialize Linda's life. Several years earlier, this facility had been named after Linda in honor of her years of service on the school board. The auditorium was filled to overflowing with people whose lives had been touched by Linda's life and educational commitment. It was a fitting place to gather to remember Linda and her legacy to the city of Akron.

By Invitation Only In certain instances, families with special concerns request that memorial services or funerals be private, by invitation only. Ginny's West Coast friends and family were concerned about her three young children and wanted a service of remembrance that would be appropriate and helpful to them. For this reason, a small invitation-only memorial and dinner were designed, focusing specifically on the children's needs. The children were encouraged to ask questions, and attendees shared stories with them. The evening was a success even though the feathers of a few friends who were left out remained a bit ruffled. All in all, the private memorial served its purpose—to positively support Ginny's grieving children.

Choir Room Remembrance Alice was in a nursing home when her husband, Norm, died. She didn't want a funeral for him. Grieving friends, however, needed to acknowledge Norm's passing, while at the same time honoring Alice's decision. They compromised by casually gathering in a place where Norm, an avid singer, had spent countless hours—the church choir room. There, on folding chairs, friends sang songs, told stories, and celebrated the life of someone they needed to remember.

No matter how you choose to remember a friend who has passed, always bear in mind the following: just as there is no single *right* way to grieve, there is no single *right* way to remember.

A DAUGHTER'S LETTER

I've known Erin since she was a little girl. Her bright red hair and shining eyes were always full of mischief. Her mother, Beth, struggled with recurring cancer for many years while facing the challenges of raising four children.

After Beth died, a mutual friend suggested Erin could use some time away, so she and her best friend flew to New York City for a short visit. There we talked about what it meant to have a mother dying of cancer, and Erin was exceptionally frank. Together we crafted her observations into this open letter to Beth's friends.

December, 2007

Dear Friends of Beth:

My mother, Beth, lived with cancer for five years. She died a year ago, leaving my dad with four children ages fifteen to twenty-nine. We are still struggling with our grief, each in our own way. There is no blueprint for how to help us through this difficult time. We simply ask you to love us through it.

My youngest brother has just started to deal with his grief. He is angry—angry at Mom for leaving him and angry because his childhood was never what it might have been. My oldest brother has a new family, with a baby born after Mom's death. As his grief finds its voice, he has the blessings of a new life to soften it. My middle brother continues his search for a new life without my mother as its center and focus.

As for me, I have worn my grief openly. My college roommates have watched me go through many phases of grieving, from isolating myself in denial, to becoming angry, and then ultimately accepting what has happened.

I want and need to remember Mom—and I do. Thank you all for letting me talk when I've needed it without constantly asking me how I'm doing. Continue to listen, even ask a question or two, but don't push me for information or resolution. It will come in its own time.

Although I know you mean well, please refrain from the tendency to try to "adopt" me. Though Mom isn't physically present, she's not gone from my life. I appreciate the occasional invitations to lunch, but I wish people would remember that I don't need a new mother.

Please hold on tightly to your memories of Mom. Don't shut them away when we're together for fear I can't deal with them. I really enjoy it when you remember and share with me the good times you experienced with Mom. It's easy to focus on that last difficult year-and-a-half instead of remembering all the good years. You can remind me of the good times.

Finally, thank you for just being there for me and my family. It has been a joy to see how many people have come back into my own life during Mom's illness and death—especially friends with whom I had lost contact. Stay in touch and we'll remember together a friend and mother who is far too precious to forget.

Love,

Erin

How Will You Remember?

There are many simple ways to remember and honor a friend's memory:

1. Write a poem or story that tells about your friendship. Consider whether to offer to share this story/poem at the funeral, save it as personal recollection for your eyes only, or to share it with select family members at a later date.
2. Set aside a special date to remember your friend each year. Many people choose their friend's birthday.
3. Gather mementos of the two of you—photographs, letters, postcards, playbills, and gifts. Keep them in a special place; peruse them whenever you want to spend time remembering your friend or mourning your loss.

Remember your friend by providing practical help for his or her grieving family.

1. Offer to handle tasks, such as donating or delivering flowers to nursing homes and shut-ins following your friend's funeral.

---

2. Offer to purchase or to help write thank-you notes for gifts and services received by the family.
3. Offer to drive older or disabled relatives to the wake, memorial service, or other memorial events and locales.

—B.

* Suggestions for this sidebar were offered by Julie Willstatter, LCSW (certified psychoanalyst, with a private practice in White Plains, New York) in conversation with the author.

Remembering Without Words

Barbara and I battled cancer together, sharing treatment milestones along with emotional ups and downs. We had become close, and now she was nearing the end of her journey. I called the hospital and asked to see her, but her family gently said no. Today wasn't a good day.

What could I do? I missed Barb and wanted—even needed—to connect with her. We had shared so much, and I felt I couldn't be totally absent in this final part of her journey.

Thinking how much we both loved Cape Cod, I picked up a paintbrush. Soon a small seascape found its way from heart to canvas, and without intending to, I spent an entire afternoon remembering Barbara as I painted.

I took the little seascape to the hospital the next week. Barb was slipping in and out of consciousness, and we were never able to share a final conversation. None-the-less, that little painting perched on the hospital windowsill spoke volumes.

When Barbara "Bluebird" Soliz died, she was buried in a Native American ceremony befitting the Mashpee Wampanoag princess that she was. Today, the little painting stands on the family mantle in remembrance of Barbara, the life she lived by the sea, and a friend who loved her dearly.

—B.

ADVOCACY AS HONOR AND REMEMBRANCE

As a friend, you may want to remember or honor someone by working as a cancer advocate. You may choose to serve as a patient advocate or participate in cancer fundraising and survivorship events.

Peg Stice works in the School of Public and Environmental Affairs at Indiana University (Indiana). She is chairperson of the Friends and Cancer board of directors and has been a long-time advocate for expanded cancer research, better cancer education, and exemplary patient care.

In the appendix, you will find the tools to advocate on behalf of a patient, researching hospitals and cancer treatments. I wanted Ms. Stice to go beyond this—to uncover other ways to advocate on behalf of friends who are cancer patients. Here are her suggestions:

Becoming a Cancer Advocate

by Peg Stice

1. **Determine individual patient's needs regarding health care systems.**

- Check to see if your friend needs or wants a professional *patient advocate.*[5] Try saying, "I've heard of something called a patient advocate. I understand they can be quite helpful in navigating the health care system. Do you have one? Would you like me to help you look into this option?"
- Ask your friend if she is aware of social services available to cancer patients through hospital or community

---

[5] The *National Cancer Institute's Dictionary of Cancer Terms* defines a patient advocate as "a person who helps a patient work with others who have an effect on the patient's health, including doctors, insurance companies, employers, case managers, and lawyers. A patient advocate helps resolve issues about health care, medical bills, and job discrimination related to a patient's medical condition." (Source: http: www. cancer.gov.)

organizations (e.g., visiting nurses, social workers). Offer to help her track down these services.

2. Be an inspiration while you advocate on behalf of cancer research, education, and policy-making. For example:

- Tell your patient-friend, "I am planning to participate in a local cancer walk-run/golf tournament and I'd like to do this in your honor. Is that okay?" If yes, carry or wear your friend's name or photo during the event; add his or her name to the list of honorees. At the event take photos to share later with your patient-friend.

- Participate with your patient-friend in cancer-related advocacy or support programs. If it's comfortable for both of you, volunteer to join your patient-friend for a Cancer Support Community (Gilda's Club or Wellness Community) activity, a community cancer event, or a cancer support program—faith-based or community-based.

- Volunteer! Fundraise! Support special cancer events; volunteer or donate to a camp for children affected by cancer. Encourage corporate philanthropy.

- Thank community leaders and business owners/managers who sponsor programs. Let them know that what they are doing matters beyond the dollars raised.[6]

- Send emails or write letters or personal notes to legislators and local leaders when you want to change something. Thank them for action. (Advocacy works—just think about how many smoke-free communities we have now.)

- Tap the power of art. Offer to record or transcribe stories shared. Encourage journaling, painting, poetry, drawing, weaving, or quilting—by the patient alone or with a group of supportive friends.[7] Offer to help your friend assemble

---

[6] See: "Making a Difference," www.cancer.net, accessed 6/15/09.

[7] Offer to find additional art resources that might be helpful and appropriate for family members including: *Sing for the Cure: Proclamation of Hope* (a CD for the Susan G. Komen Foundation); *Just Stand Up (Artists Stand Up to Cancer); Artists-In-Residence: The Creative Center's Approach to Arts in Healthcare* (www.thecreativecenter.org.).

an album or scrapbook of cards and letters received during diagnosis and recovery.

- Think PINK. (Or not.) Wearing ribbons or T-shirts and buying cause-related marketing products raises much needed funds and can contribute to a strong feeling of unity. There are critics, however, who look at this marketing strategy from a different perspective.[8] It's up to you!

- Don't be surprised if your survivor becomes a self-advocate for better cancer care and awareness.[9] If this happens, volunteer to coordinate his or her speaking engagements, to publicize events, or to distribute literature. Be creative and get others involved.

- Contact local nonprofit organizations or a university civic engagement office. If the university offers nonprofit management classes, see if your idea for fundraising or a research project might be a good match for service-learning projects. Students may be willing to help you with planning special events, research, grant writing, etc.

The opportunities to advocate on behalf of people with cancer are limited only by the extent of your creativity, commitment, time, and energy. It means going the extra mile on behalf of patient-friends to help them secure the best medical care available. It means helping to raise funds for cancer research or to promote cancer awareness and prevention. From self-advocacy to collaborative efforts that promote teamwork, challenge or change attitudes/policies/practices, advocates "give voice" to this important cause.

A SPECIAL REMEMBRANCE

Jessica Bechhofer is a college student. She and David Bechhofer are a Massachusetts father-daughter cancer-activist team. David is responsible for creating the Susan G. Komen 3-Day Youth Corps

---

[8] Samantha King, *Pink Ribbons, Inc.: Breast Cancer and the Politics of Philanthropy*, Minneapolis: University of Minnesota Press, 2006.

[9] See *Self-Advocacy: A Cancer Survivor's Handbook* (Silver Spring, MD: National Coalition for Cancer Survivorship, 2009).

and the Avon Walk for Breast Cancer Youth Crew. Here are their thoughts on becoming cancer activists:

Jessica and David

by Jessica and David Bechhofer

Jessica

I began my journey as a cancer activist at age five, when my father and I participated in a breast cancer walk in Boston. I held up a sign that said, "My mommy died, but I want to live!"

Two years later I began working as a volunteer on the (Avon) Boston Breast Cancer 3-Day walk. At thirteen, I helped my father create the Boston 3-Day Youth Corps, a group of teens affected by breast cancer. These were teens who wanted to make a difference. For three years, I teamed with those kids working on the 3-Day crew until, at sixteen, I was finally allowed to walk in the event with three friends. By moving from volunteer to participant, I took the next step along my personal path of cancer activism.

The signs I held up, the T-shirts I wore, and the events in which I participated have allowed me to share my story. Activism renewed my sense of purpose, even as I mourned the loss of my mother.

David

Jessica's mother, my first wife, Suzanne, died at age thirty-five. In her last days, Suzanne expressed a fear that as our lives went on, she would be forgotten. Our activism has served multiple purposes:

- It keeps our memory of Suzanne bright.
- It channels our grief and loss into something constructive.
- In the face of death, it reaffirms life.

In 2002, Jessica was invited to speak to the participants on the Breast Cancer 3-Day walk held in Boston. I told her that this was her opportunity to tell our family's story and I would help draft it. So one spring evening at a campsite in front of three thousand people, young Jessica delivered her speech. She said in part,

> I am ten years old. My mom was diagnosed with breast cancer when she was pregnant with me. She fought very hard against the disease but died when I was three and a half.
>
> I got a new mom three years ago. She walked in the first Boston 3-Day, crewed last year, and is walking again this year. I am very proud of her. Today I'm wearing a T-shirt that says,

**"I'm working on the 3-Day.
In memory of one mom. In support of another."**

Jessica's passion and commitment became the example that spawned the creation of the Boston Breast Cancer 3-Day Youth Corps, two years later. Her advocacy and activism efforts helped Jessica to focus her energy on something positive—to continue fighting for the advances in cancer treatment and care, and to show others what they can do to honor the loved one they want to remember.

A FINAL QUESTION

As you share gifts of friendship—from hope and delight, to peace and remembrance—a final question arises: In the enormity of my friend's cancer experience, can my gift of friendship really make a difference? The answer is a resounding "Yes!" Every expression of friendship during cancer, whether in word or deed, is a message from the heart that says, "You are not alone; you are traveling in the company of a friend." The contributors to this book commend each of you, our readers and friends, for stepping forward to share in another's cancer journey. We sincerely wish you times of healing, the many gifts of friendship, and Godspeed as you travel together, friend-to-friend.

—Bonnie Draeger

ACKNOWLEDGMENTS

To the many contributors to this book:
You donated your time and shared your experiences and expertise
to educate friends of people with cancer. Words cannot express the
depth of my gratitude for your generosity and encouragement. The
impact of your gifts of knowledge will be felt for years to come.
Thank you!

To those who inspired our work and enabled our vision,
this book would not have been possible without you.

Michael Abram

Suzanne Bechhofer

Barbara Ann Bell

Lin M. Bradley

Nooy Bunnell

Debbie Bushfield

Carol Campbell

Nancy Campbell

Helene Cantarelle

Cynthia Chapman

Marilyn Cook

Dorothy Draeger

Wayne Draeger

Isobel Fisher

Saul Fisher

Moriah Fowler

Inge Opsomer Giltay

Zachary Todd Jemison

Beth Jensen

Barbara Johnson

Rosanne Kalick

Bill Levin

Cameron Riley McClain

John M. McClure

Cynthia Northrup

Julia Papper

Kathleen Reinke

Michal Rubin

George Russell

Regina Ryan

Lois Sadogierski

Lynn Shonk

Diane Simpler

Bill Stice

Suzie Snavely

Joseph Sverchek

Barbara Soliz

Fran Stone

Doris Spence

William T. Webb

Hazel Wendt

Susan Wendt

William Wendt

Karen Winkel

Ruth Zie

And with special appreciation to the Board of Directors
Friends & Cancer (In Marjolein's Memory, Inc.)
and
Margaret "Peg" Stice, Chairperson
for your decade of tireless efforts and unending support
on behalf of this project.

To all of you and the countless others who have
contributed to this book in so many ways,
"Thank You!"

Appendix

RESOURCES FOR RESEARCHING CANCER INFORMATION, CANCER TREATMENTS, AND CANCER CENTERS

In this appendix you will find a host of cancer resources readily available to patients and their friends. If you have only a little time to research basic information or cancer treatment facilities, here is a "short list" of several top cancer websites.

This appendix also includes information on how to evaluate additional websites from journalist, web designer, and webmaster, Gena Asher. Finally, there is a list of recommended books and over forty-five websites offering information on specific cancers and cancer-related topics.

General Information: Cancer and
Cancer Treatment Centers

National Institutes of Health

This U.S. government organization provides comprehensive and up-to-date cancer information. Their websites (www.cancer.gov and www.nlm.nih.gov/medlineplus) are your first stop for cancer information on all types of cancer, cancer treatments, and cancer treatment facilities.

National Cancer Institute
800-4-CANCER or 800-422-6237
www.cancer.gov

NCI lists sixteen *cancer centers* and forty *comprehensive cancer centers*. NCI-designated comprehensive cancer centers integrate leading cancer research with patient services such as clinical care, education, and outreach. They provide free booklets (online and printed), "fact sheets" for specific cancers and cancer-related topics, information on clinical trials, and much more.

Medline Plus
www.nlm.nih.gov/medlineplus

Information on any form of cancer can be obtained by accessing the National Institute of Health's "medline." (Hint: After locating the website, click on "health topics" and select "cancers.")

National Comprehensive Cancer Network
215-T690-0300
www.nccn.com

This organization's website provides direct links to each of twenty-one leading cancer centers (e.g., Memorial Sloan-Kettering Cancer Center, M.D. Anderson Cancer Center, City of Hope Comprehensive Cancer Center). It is especially useful for researching various cancer centers' specialties and clinical trials. (Hint: Click on "NCCN Member Institutions" and choose a specific institution you'd like to research.)

Cancer*Care*

800-813-4673

www.cancercare.org

For over sixty years, Cancer*Care* has provided professional support for anyone affected by cancer free of charge. These free services include: professional counseling by oncology social workers, financial assistance, workshops, support groups, online cancer resources, booklets, and factsheets.

American Cancer Society

800-227-2345

www.cancer.org

This well-known cancer organization's website provides information on cancer basics/treatments/side effects/cancer-related topics, specifics on over seventy types of cancer, a glossary of terms, and more. Free materials can be ordered or downloaded directly.

Cancer.Net

888-651-3038

www.cancer.net

The American Society of Clinical Oncology's website offers easily understood fact sheets for adult and childhood cancers, cancer treatments, and treatment side effects. (Hint: go to the "site map" and type in *ASCO Answers fact sheet* to locate your topic.)

THE WEB AS FRIEND OR FOE

The Internet is alive with cancer websites—some helpful and others not. How do you know which information to trust? To help us know how to evaluate websites for specific cancers and cancer-related topics, I turned to Gena Asher.

I met Ms. Asher shortly after she was honored for her outstanding website development by the Woman's Press Club of Indiana. She is the founder and Webmaster for BreastCancerFYI.org, a website created especially for Indiana breast cancer patients and survivors. Ms. Asher is a cancer survivor. She teaches at the Indiana University School of Journalism where she is the Web editor. Here are Ms. Asher's tips on searching the Web for credible cancer information:

USING THE INTERNET RESPONSIBLY

by Gena Asher

Of all people in crisis, cancer patients may be most likely to grab at urban legends, pseudo-science, and outright misinformation. Fear often overtakes their usual good sense, and it may be a friend's duty to steer them away from junk science and toward the multitudes of useful, authoritative resources on the Internet or in printed materials.

Shortly after my breast cancer diagnosis, a friend forwarded an e-mail to me that outlined a recipe for "Cancer Curing Soup." This antioxidant-rich concoction promised to eradicate those pesky cancer cells better than chemo, radiation, or any pharmaceutical potion.

A few weeks later, I visited a support group where participants shared cancer experiences, lessons, and advice. There an eager participant clutched a sheaf of printouts as though they were the Holy Grail. She began to talk about a "secret" potion that Native Canadians had proved would cure cancer. She claimed one pharmaceutical company knew all about it but couldn't patent it and therefore would not develop it.

While the soup was quite tasty, the tale of the secret potion disturbed me. I vowed to be wary of anyone—or anything—touting unsubstantiated claims of a cure for cancer.

Information is powerful. However, one must *always* evaluate the quality of that information. If that duty falls to you, you will first want to consider the following suggestions for assessing the quality of a source or website information. You also will want to be highly sensitive to your friend's "information tolerance level."

When You've Been Asked to Gather Information: Tolerance Levels

Cancer patients may want your help in finding as much data as possible about a certain drug or procedure, but may turn away when you present them with a stack of printed pages. Some days, information overload makes managing the disease seem insurmountable and the medical jargon overwhelming. It may be up to you to read great amounts of information, gather details from doctors, and then somehow give your friend the *Readers Digest* version!

Other friends may not want your help at all, as was the case for a friend of mine. She was distressed because her aunt refused to hear any details about her recurrent cancer. She wouldn't even ask her medical team questions. Some patients may be distressed to read the often dismal survival statistics or treatment options. Others simply rely on what the medical professionals tell them, without question or additional information. While this is hard for many caring friends to accept, we all have different tolerance levels for information, especially when that information may be frightening.

Evaluating Internet Information

As you research Internet sites for reliable information, it is important to ask the following questions:

- Is the site selling something?
- Am I looking at an institution's document or an individual's?
- Are the following reliable extensions found in the Internet address: .gov, .org, .mil, or .edu?

   This is not to say ".com" and ".net" aren't reputable, but they may be commercial enterprises or laypersons' information. *Use these for background and general knowledge.* You may pick up on a thread of info that you can research in more authoritative sites later.

- When was the site updated?

  In cancer research, updates and protocols change quickly. If a site was last updated two or more years ago, use it as background research but continue looking for more recent information on that topic.

- Is there someone to contact?

  Who is responsible for this site? It may be a nonprofit agency such as the American Cancer Society or a medical organization such as a local hospital, but someone should be accountable for the information on the site. Look for phone numbers, names, and physical addresses in addition to e-mail addresses.

- Is the information accurate? Does it seem in sync with what you are hearing from medical practitioners? Does it have any "stamp of approval?"

  Some organizations, such as Health on the Net, allow websites that conform to its standards to post its special icon. Check the "About Us" page for more information, and be wary of sites that do not have "About Us" as a link.

- Does the information cite sources that you can verify?

  Using a simple Google search, you can cross-check information presented on websites to see if there are other sources for it. Reputable sites such as Cancer.gov may link to other sources. In these cases, you can be reasonably sure that Cancer.gov won't link to junk science websites and that it extends its authority to its links.

Evaluations aside, some information is decidedly unprofessional, but still may offer ideas that could be useful to patients and caregivers. Forums and chats include postings from cancer patients who often compare notes on treatments and treatment side effects. The danger here is in regarding these sites as "medical advice."

"Your friend should be cautioned about the use of Internet chat rooms discussing procedures or physicians," says Joseph Disa, MD, Memorial Sloan-Kettering Cancer Center. "These may only serve to unnecessarily heighten anxiety prior to a procedure or even provide misinformation."[84]

Always remind patient-friends that these sites are not intended to replace sound medical counsel. In truth, they are akin to *support groups*—people out there sharing the same experience, whether as patients, family members, or friends.

WEBSITES FOR SPECIFIC CANCERS AND CANCER-RELATED TOPICS

All websites listed in this section meet the criterion established by Friends & Cancer. This criterion is a compilation of that proposed by Ms. Asher, with additional criterion recommended by the American Library Association, and/or the National Endowment for the Humanities:

1. Each website must represent a reputable, not-for-profit foundation, 501(c)(3) organization, medical professionals' organization, hospital, or government public health service organization, providing cancer information, services, and/or patient-family support.

2. The website must contain free, authoritative cancer information for patients, or patients' families and friends, and may include additional information specifically for cancer care professionals.

3. The website must be easy to navigate, with information readily accessible, and may include links to other well regarded cancer information sites.

4. The website must include complete contact information along with general information on the sponsoring organization, its mission, and its services.

---

[84] Dr. Joseph Disa, MD, New York, New York, in correspondence with Bonnie Draeger.

Alternative Medicine (*see* Complementary Integrative Medicine)

Bladder Cancer

Bladder Cancer Advocacy Network
  www.bcan.org
AUA Foundation
  www.urologyhealth.org

Bone Cancer

The Bone and Cancer Foundation
  www.boneandcancerfoundation.org

Bone Marrow/Stem Cell Transplant

National Bone Marrow Transplant Link
  http://nbmtlink.org

Brain Cancer

American Brain Tumor Association
  www.abta.org
National Brain Tumor Foundation
  www.braintumor.org

Breast Cancer

Breastcancer.org
  www.breastcancer.org
Susan G. Komen for the Cure
  www.komen.org

Caregiving

Cleaning for a Reason
  www.cleaningforareason.org

National Alliance for Caregiving
    www.caregiving.org

Cervical Cancer (*see* Gynecologic Cancers)

Chemotherapy
Chemocare.com
    www.chemocare.com

Children's Cancers (*see* Pediatric Cancers)

Clinical Trials

ClinicalTrials.gov
    www.clinicaltrials.gov
National Comprehensive Cancer Network
    www.nccn.com

Colorectal Cancer

Colon Cancer Alliance
    www.ccalliance.org

Communication

CaringBridge
    www.caringbridge.org

Complementary Integrative Medicine

National Center for Complementary and Alternative Medicine
    www.nccam.nih.gov

Finance, Insurance and Workplace Issues

National Coalition for Cancer Survivorship
    www.canceradvocacy.org
Cancer*Care*
    www.cancercare.org

Gynecologic Cancers

Women's Cancer Network
    www.wcn.org

Hodgkin's Disease (*see* Lymphoma)

Hospice

Hospice Foundation of America
    www.hospicefoundation.org

Housing Assistance

Ronald McDonald House Charities
    www.rmhc.org

Kidney Cancer

American Urological Association Foundation
    www.urologyhealth.org
Kidney Cancer Association
    www.KidneyCancer.org

Leukemia

Leukemia & Lymphoma Society
    www.lls.org

Liver Cancer

American Liver Foundation
    www.liverfoundation.org

Lung Cancer

American Lung Association
    www.lung.org
Cancer*Care*
    www.lungcancer.org

Lung Cancer Alliance
www.alcase.org

Lymphomas

Leukemia & Lymphoma Society
www.lls.org

Multiple Myeloma

International Myeloma Foundation
www.myeloma.org

Nutrition

Oncolink
www.oncolink.org

Ovarian Cancer (*see also* Gynecologic Cancers)

Women's Cancer Network
www.wcn.org
National Ovarian Cancer Coalition
www.ovarian.org
Ovarian Cancer National Alliance
www.ovariancancer.org

Pancreatic Cancer

Pancreatic Cancer Action Network
www.pancan.org

Patient Advocacy (*see also* specific cancers)

National Coalition for Cancer Survivorship
www.canceradvocacy.org

Pediatric Cancers

Children's Cancer Research
www.childrenscancer.org

National Children's Cancer Society
   www.thenccs.org

Prostate Cancer

American Urological Association Foundation
   www.urologyhealth.org
Prostate Conditions Education Council
   www.prostateconditions.org

Radiation Therapy

RadiologyInfo.org
   www.radiologyinfo.org

Support Programs

Cancer Support Community
   www.cancersupportcommunity.org
SuperSibs (for siblings of pediatric cancer patients)
   www.supersibs.org
I'm Too Young For This! (for young adults)
   www.Imtooyoungforthis.org

Survivorship

National Coalition for Cancer Survivorship
   www.canceradvocacy.org

Testicular Cancer

American Urological Association Foundation
   www.urologyhealth.org

Thyroid Cancer

ThyCa: Thyroid Cancer Survivors' Association, Inc.
   www.thyca.org

Transportation Assistance

Air Charity Network
www.aircharitynetwork.org

Uterine Cancer (*see* Gynecologic Cancers)

FURTHER READING

100 Questions and Answers About™ *[cancer] series.* Sudbury, MA: Jones and Bartlett Publishers.

Babcock, Elise NeeDell. *When Life Becomes Precious: The Essential Guide for Patients, Loved Ones, and Friends of Those Facing Serious Illnesses.* New York: Bantam, 2002. Reissue of New York: Bantam, 1997.

Beavers, Brett and Tom Douglas. *Something Worth Leaving Behind.* Nashville: Rutledge Hill Press, 2002.

Clark, Elizabeth. *You Have the Right to Be Hopeful,* 2nd ed. Silver Spring, MD: National Coalition for Cancer Survivorship, 1999.

Girard, Vickie. *There's No Place Like Hope: A Guide to Beating Cancer in Mind-Sized Bites,* Dan Zadra, ed. Lynnwood, Wash.: Compendium, Inc., 2004.

Halpern, Susan P. *The Etiquette of Illness.* New York: Bloomsbury, 2004.

Harpham, Wendy Schlessel. *When a Parent Has Cancer: A Guide to Caring for Your Children.* New York: Perennial Currents, 2004. First published by Harper-Collins Publishers in 1997.

Holland, Jimmie C. and Sheldon Lewis. *The Human Side of Cancer: Living with Hope, Coping with Uncertainty.* New York: Quill, 2001.

Kalick, Rosanne. *Cancer Etiquette: What to Say, What to Do, When Someone You Know or Love Has Cancer.* Scarsdale, NY: Lion Books, 2005.

Katz, Rebecca with Mat Edelson. *The Cancer-Fighting Kitchen: Nourishing, Big-Flavor Recipes for Cancer Treatment and Recovery.* Berkeley: Celestial Arts, 2009.

National Cancer Institute. *What You Need to Know About™ [cancer]* series. Bethesda: National Cancer Institute, 1994–2003.

Orchard, Anne. *Their Cancer—Your Journey: A Traveller's Guide for Carers, Family and Friends.* Charmouth, Bridport, UK: Rainbow Heart Publishing, 2008.

Rose, Susannah L. and Richard T. Hara. *100 Questions and Answers About Caring for Family or Friends with Cancer.* Sudbury, MA: Jones and Bartlett Publishers, 2005.

Rosenbaum, Ernest H. and Isadora Rosenbaum. *Everyone's Guide to Cancer Supportive Care: A Comprehensive Handbook for Patients and Their Families.* Kansas City, MO: Andrews McMeel, 2005.

Sheehy, Gail. *Passages In Caregiving: Turning Chaos into Confidence.* New York: William Morrow (HarperCollins), 2010.

Smith, Harold Ivan. *Grieving the Death of a Friend.* Minneapolis: Augsburg Fortress, 1996.

GLOSSARY

When cancer strikes, everyday conversations between friends become more complicated. There are so many unfamiliar terms and expressions. While it is not necessary to learn all the terms listed here, it is important to be able to access their definitions when your patient-friend mentions them in conversation.

Librarian and cancer survivor, Lonny Fleishman, has prepared this glossary of common cancer terms you are likely to encounter. The definitions below are excerpted directly from the National Cancer Institute's *Dictionary of Cancer Terms* (http://www.cancer.gov/dictionary).

acute—Symptoms or signs that begin and worsen quickly; not chronic.

adenoma—A tumor that is not cancer. It starts in gland-like cells of the epithelial tissue (thin layer of tissue that covers organs, glands, and other structures within the body).

adjunct therapy—Another treatment used together with the primary treatment. Its purpose is to assist the primary treatment. Also called adjunctive therapy.

adjuvant therapy—Additional cancer treatment given after the primary treatment to lower the risk that the cancer will come back. Adjuvant therapy may include chemotherapy, radiation therapy, hormone therapy, targeted therapy, or biological therapy.

advance directive—A legal document that states the treatment or care a person wishes to receive or not receive if he or she becomes unable to make medical decisions (for example, due to being unconscious or in a coma). Some types of advance directives are living wills and do-not-resuscitate (DNR) orders.

angiogenesis inhibitor—A substance that may prevent the formation of blood vessels. In anticancer therapy, an angiogenesis inhibitor may prevent the growth of new blood vessels that tumors need to grow.

benign—Not cancerous. Benign tumors may grow larger but do not spread to other parts of the body. Also called nonmalignant.

biological therapy—Treatment to boost or restore the ability of the immune system to fight cancer, infections, and other diseases. Also used to lessen certain side effects that may be caused by some cancer treatments. Agents used in biological therapy include monoclonal antibodies, growth factors, and vaccines. These agents may also have a direct antitumor effect. Also called biological response modifier therapy, biotherapy, BRM therapy. and immunotherapy.

biomarker—A biological molecule found in blood, other body fluids, or tissues that is a sign of a normal or abnormal process, or of a condition or disease. A biomarker may be used to see how well the body responds to a treatment for a disease or condition. Also called molecular marker and signature molecule.

biopsy—The removal of cells or tissues for examination by a pathologist. The pathologist may study the tissue under a microscope or perform other tests on the cells or tissue. There are many different types of biopsy procedures.

bone marrow transplantation—A procedure to replace bone marrow that has been destroyed by treatment with high doses of anticancer drugs or radiation. Transplantation may be autologous (an individual's own marrow saved before treatment), allogeneic (marrow donated by someone else), or syngeneic (marrow donated by an identical twin).

cancer—A term for diseases in which abnormal cells divide without control and can invade nearby tissues. Cancer cells can also spread to other parts of the body through the blood and lymph systems. There are several main types of cancer. Carcinoma is cancer that begins in the skin or in tissues that line or cover internal organs. Sarcoma is a cancer that begins in bone, cartilage, fat, muscle, blood vessels, or other connective or supportive tissue. Leukemia is a cancer that starts in blood-forming tissue such as the bone marrow, and causes large numbers of abnormal blood cells to be produced and enter the blood. Lymphoma and multiple myeloma are cancers that begin in the cells of the immune system. Central nervous system cancers are cancers that begin in the tissues of the brain and spinal cord. Also called malignancy.

Cancer Information Service (CIS)—The Cancer Information Service is the National Cancer Institute's link to the public, interpreting and explaining research findings in a clear and understandable manner, and providing personalized responses to specific questions about cancer. Access the CIS by calling 1-800-4-CANCER (1-800-422-6237), or by using the LiveHelp instant-messaging service at https://livehelp.cancer.gov.

carcinogen—Any substance that causes cancer.

carcinogenesis—The process by which normal cells are transformed into cancer cells.

carcinoma—Cancer that begins in the skin or in tissues that line or cover internal organs.

CAT scan [CT scan]—A series of detailed pictures of areas inside the body taken from different angles. The pictures are created by a computer linked to an x-ray machine. Also called computed tomography scan, computerized axial tomography scan, and computerized tomography, and CT scan.

CBC—A test to check the number of red blood cells, white blood cells, and platelets in a sample of blood. Also called blood cell count and complete blood count.

chronic—A disease or condition that persists or progresses over a long period of time.

clinical trial—A type of research study that tests how well new medical approaches work in people. These studies test new methods of screening, prevention, diagnosis, or treatment of a disease. Also called clinical study.

combination chemotherapy—Treatment using more than one anticancer drug.

complete remission—The disappearance of all signs of cancer in response to treatment. This does not always mean the cancer has been cured. Also called complete response.

cyst—A sac or capsule in the body. It may be filled with fluid or other material.

differentiation—In cancer, refers to how mature (developed) the cancer cells are in a tumor. Differentiated tumor cells resemble normal cells and tend to grow and spread at a slower rate than undifferentiated or poorly differentiated tumor cells, which lack the structure and function of normal cells and grow uncontrollably.

dysplasia—Cells that look abnormal under a microscope but are not cancer.

first-line therapy—Initial treatment used to reduce a cancer. First-line therapy is followed by other treatments such as chemotherapy, radiation therapy, and hormone therapy to get rid of cancer that remains. Also called induction therapy, primary therapy, and primary treatment.

gene—The functional and physical unit of heredity passed from parent to offspring. Genes are pieces of DNA, and most genes contain the information for making a specific protein.

gene therapy—A type of experimental treatment in which foreign genetic material (DNA or RNA) is inserted into a person's cells to prevent or fight disease. Gene therapy is being studied in the treatment of certain types of cancer.

genetic marker—Alteration in DNA that may indicate an increased risk of developing a specific disease or disorder.

genetic testing—Analyzing DNA to look for a genetic alteration that may indicate an increased risk for developing a specific disease or disorder.

grading—A system for classifying cancer cells in terms of how abnormal they appear when examined under a microscope. The objective of a grading system is to provide information about the probable growth rate of the tumor and its tendency to spread. The systems used to grade tumors vary with each type of cancer. Grading plays a role in treatment decisions.

hemoglobin—The substance inside red blood cells that binds to oxygen in the lungs and carries it to the tissues.

high-dose chemotherapy—An intensive drug treatment to kill cancer cells, but that also destroys the bone marrow and can cause other severe side effects. High-dose chemotherapy is usually followed by bone marrow or stem cell transplantation to rebuild the bone marrow.

high-dose radiation—An amount of radiation that is greater than that given in typical radiation therapy. High-dose radiation is precisely directed at the tumor to avoid damaging healthy tissue, and may kill more cancer cells in fewer treatments. Also called HDR.

hospice—A program that provides special care for people who are near the end of life and for their families, either at home, in freestanding facilities, or within hospitals.

hyperplasia—An abnormal increase in the number of normal cells in an organ or tissue.

hyperthermia therapy—A type of treatment in which body tissue is exposed to high temperatures to damage and kill cancer cells or to make cancer cells more sensitive to the effects of radiation and certain anticancer drugs.

imaging—In medicine, a process that makes pictures of areas inside the body. Imaging uses methods such as x-rays (high-energy radiation), ultrasound (high-energy sound waves), and radio waves.

implant radiation therapy—A type of radiation therapy in which radioactive material sealed in needles, seeds, wires, or catheters is placed directly into or near a tumor. Also called brachytherapy, internal radiation therapy, and radiation brachytherapy.

infusion—A method of putting fluids, including drugs, into the bloodstream. Also called intravenous infusion.

invasive cancer—Cancer that has spread beyond the layer of tissue in which it developed and is growing into surrounding, healthy tissues. Also called infiltrating cancer.

invasive procedure—A medical procedure that invades (enters) the body, usually by cutting or puncturing the skin or by inserting instruments into the body.

laser therapy—Treatment that uses intense, narrow beams of light to cut and destroy tissue, such as cancer tissue. Laser therapy may also be used to reduce lymphedema (swelling caused by a buildup of lymph fluid in tissue) after breast cancer surgery.

late-stage cancer—A term used to describe cancer that is far along in its growth, and has spread to the lymph nodes or other places in the body.

lymph node—A rounded mass of lymphatic tissue that is surrounded by a capsule of connective tissue. Lymph nodes filter lymph (lymphatic fluid), and they store lymphocytes (white blood cells). They are located along lymphatic vessels. Also called lymph gland.

lymphedema—A condition in which extra lymph fluid builds up in tissues and causes swelling. It may occur in an arm or leg if lymph vessels are blocked, damaged, or removed by surgery.

malignant—Cancerous. Malignant cells can invade and destroy nearby tissue and spread to other parts of the body.

mammogram—An x-ray of the breast.

margin—The edge or border of the tissue removed in cancer surgery. The margin is described as negative or clean when the pathologist finds no cancer cells at the edge of the tissue, suggesting that all of the cancer has been removed. The margin is described as positive or involved when the pathologist finds cancer cells at the edge of the tissue, suggesting that all of the cancer has not been removed.

medical oncologist—A doctor who specializes in diagnosing and treating cancer using chemotherapy, hormonal therapy, biological therapy, and targeted therapy. A medical oncologist often is the main health care provider for someone who has cancer. A medical oncologist also gives supportive care and may coordinate treatment given by other specialists.

metastasis—The spread of cancer from one part of the body to another. A tumor formed by cells that have spread is called a "metastatic tumor" or a "metastasis." The metastatic tumor contains cells that are like those in the original (primary) tumor. The plural form of metastasis is metastases.

modality—A method of treatment. For example, surgery and chemotherapy are treatment modalities.

MRI—A procedure in which radio waves and a powerful magnet linked to a computer are used to create detailed pictures of areas inside the body. These pictures can show the difference between normal and diseased tissue. MRI makes better images of organs and soft tissue than other scanning techniques, such as computed tomography (CT) or x-ray. MRI is especially useful for imaging the brain, the spine, the soft tissue of joints, and the inside of bones. Also called magnetic resonance imaging, NMRI, and nuclear magnetic resonance imaging.

neoadjuvant therapy—Treatment given as a first step to shrink a tumor before the main treatment, which is usually surgery, is given. Examples of neoadjuvant therapy include chemotherapy, radiation therapy, and hormone therapy.

neoplasm—An abnormal mass of tissue that results when cells divide more than they should or do not die when they should. Neoplasms may be benign (not cancerous), or malignant (cancerous). Also called tumor.

neuropathy—A nerve problem that causes pain, numbness, tingling, swelling, or muscle weakness in different parts of the body. It usually begins in the hands or feet and gets worse over time. Neuropathy may be caused by physical injury, infection, toxic substances, disease (such as cancer, diabetes, kidney failure, or malnutrition), or drugs, including anticancer drugs. Also called peripheral neuropathy.

nodule—A growth or lump that may be malignant (cancer) or benign (not cancer).

noninvasive—In medicine, it describes a procedure that does not require inserting an instrument through the skin or into a body opening. In cancer, it describes disease that has not spread outside the tissue in which it began.

nuclear grade—An evaluation of the size and shape of the nucleus in tumor cells and the percentage of tumor cells that are in the process of dividing or growing. Cancers with low nuclear grade grow and spread less quickly than cancers with high nuclear grade.

oncologist—A doctor who specializes in treating cancer. Some oncologists specialize in a particular type of cancer treatment. For example, a radiation oncologist specializes in treating cancer with radiation.

oncology—The study of cancer.

palliative care—Care given to improve the quality of life of patients who have a serious or life-threatening disease. The goal of palliative care is to prevent or treat as early as possible the symptoms of a disease, side effects caused by treatment of a disease, and psychological, social, and spiritual problems related to a disease or its treatment. Also called comfort care, supportive care, and symptom management.

pathologist—A doctor who identifies diseases by studying cells and tissues under a microscope.

pathology report—The description of cells and tissues made by a pathologist based on microscopic evidence, and sometimes used to make a diagnosis of a disease.

patient advocate—A person who helps a patient work with others who have an effect on the patient's health, including doctors, insurance companies, employers, case managers, and lawyers. A patient advocate helps resolve issues about health care, medical bills, and job discrimination related to a patient's medical condition. Cancer advocacy groups try to raise public awareness about important cancer issues, such as the need for cancer support services, education, and research. Such groups work to bring about change that will help cancer patients and their families.

PCA—A method of pain relief in which the patient controls the amount of pain medicine that is used. When pain relief is needed, the person can receive a preset dose of pain medicine by pressing a button on a computerized pump that is connected to a small tube in the body. Also called patient-controlled analgesia.

PET scan—A procedure in which a small amount of radioactive glucose (sugar) is injected into a vein, and a scanner is used to make detailed, computerized pictures of areas inside the body where the glucose is used. Because cancer cells often use more glucose than normal cells, the pictures can be used to find cancer cells in the body. Also called positron emission tomography scan.

photodynamic therapy—Treatment with drugs that become active when exposed to light. These activated drugs may kill cancer cells.

port—An implanted device through which blood may be withdrawn and drugs may be infused without repeated needle sticks. Also called port-a-cath.

radiation therapy—The use of high-energy radiation from x-rays, gamma rays, neutrons, protons, and other sources to kill cancer cells and shrink tumors. Radiation may come from a machine outside the body (external-beam radiation therapy), or it may come from radioactive material placed in the body near cancer cells (internal radiation therapy). Systemic radiation therapy uses a radioactive substance, such as a radiolabeled monoclonal antibody, that travels in the blood to tissues throughout the body. Also called irradiation and radiotherapy.

remission—A decrease in or disappearance of signs and symptoms of cancer. In partial remission, some, but not all, signs and symptoms of cancer have disappeared. In complete remission, all signs and symptoms of cancer have disappeared, although cancer still may be in the body.

sentinel lymph node biopsy—Removal and examination of the sentinel node(s) (the first lymph node(s) to which cancer cells are likely to spread from a primary tumor). To identify the sentinel lymph node(s), the surgeon injects a radioactive substance, blue dye, or both near the tumor. The surgeon then uses a probe to find the sentinel lymph node(s) containing the radioactive substance or looks for the lymph node(s) stained with dye. The surgeon then removes the sentinel node(s) to check for the presence of cancer cells.

serum tumor marker test—A blood test that measures the amount of substances called tumor markers (or biomarkers). Tumor markers are released into the blood by tumor cells or by other cells in response to tumor cells. A high level of a tumor marker may be a sign of cancer.

sonogram—A computer picture of areas inside the body created by bouncing high-energy sound waves (ultrasound) off internal tissues or organs. Also called ultrasonogram.

stage—The extent of a cancer in the body. Staging is usually based on the size of the tumor, whether lymph nodes contain cancer, and whether the cancer has spread from the original site to other parts of the body. (Ed. Note: For information on the stages of specific cancers, access cancer.gov/dictionary: Stage 0, Stage I, Stage II, Stage III, or Stage IV.)

staging—Performing exams and tests to learn the extent of the cancer within the body, especially whether the disease has spread from the original site to other parts of the body. It is important to know the stage of the disease in order to plan the best treatment.

targeted therapy—A type of treatment that uses drugs or other substances, such as monoclonal antibodies, to identify and attack specific cancer cells. Targeted therapy may have fewer side effects than other types of cancer treatments.

tumor—An abnormal mass of tissue that results when cells divide more than they should or do not die when they should. Tumors may be benign (not cancerous), or malignant (cancerous). Also called neoplasm.

tumor marker—A substance found in tissue, blood, or other body fluids that may be a sign of cancer or certain benign (non-cancerous) conditions. Most tumor markers are made by both normal cells and cancer cells, but they are made in larger amounts by cancer cells. A tumor marker may help to diagnose cancer, plan treatment, or find out how well treatment is working, or if cancer has come back. Examples of tumor markers include CA-125 (in ovarian cancer), CA 15-3 (in breast cancer), CEA (in colon cancer), and PSA (in prostate cancer).

ultrasound—A procedure in which high-energy sound waves are bounced off internal tissues or organs and make echoes. The echo patterns are shown on the screen of an ultrasound machine, forming a picture of body tissues called a sonogram. Also called ultrasonography.

undifferentiated—A term used to describe cells or tissues that do not have specialized ("mature") structures or functions. Undifferentiated cancer cells often grow and spread quickly.

WBC—A type of immune cell. Most WBCs are made in the bone marrow and are found in the blood and lymph tissue. WBCs help the body fight infections and other diseases. Granulocytes, monocytes, and lymphocytes are WBCs. Also called leukocyte and white blood cell.

wide local excision—Surgery to cut out the cancer and some healthy tissue around it.

BIBLIOGRAPHY

Babcock, Elise NeeDell. *When Life Becomes Precious: The Essential Guide for Patients, Loved Ones, and Friends of Those Facing Serious Illnesses.* New York: Bantam, 2002. Reissue of New York: Bantam, 1997.

Beavers, Brett and Tom Douglas. *Something Worth Leaving Behind.* Nashville: Rutledge Hill Press, 2002.

Clark, Elizabeth J. *You Have the Right to Be Hopeful,* 2nd ed. Silver Spring, MD: National Coalition for Cancer Survivorship, 1999.

Cousins, Norman. *Anatomy of an Illness.* New York: W.W. Norton & Company, Inc., 1979.

Drescher, Fran. *Cancer Schmancer.* New York: Warner Books, 2002.

Girard, Vickie. *There's No Place Like Hope: A Guide to Beating Cancer in Mind-Sized Bites.* Ed. Dan Zadra. Lynnwood, WA: Compendium, Inc., 2004.

Greive, Bradley Trevor. *The Blue Day Book: A Lesson in Cheering Yourself Up.* Kansas City, Mo.: Andrews McMeel, 2000.

Hanh, Thich Nhat. *Peace is Every Step: The Path of Mindfulness in Everyday Life.* New York: Bantam Books, 1992.

With special appreciation to Carol Tsang, PhD, who prepared the initial bibliography.

Hanh, Thich Nhat. *The Miracle of Mindfulness: An Introduction to the Practice of Meditation.* Translated by Mobi Ho. Boston: Beacon Press, 1987.

Halpern, Susan P. *The Etiquette of Illness.* New York: Bloomsbury, 2004.

Harpham, Wendy Schlessel. *When a Parent Has Cancer: A Guide to Caring for Your Children.* New York: Perennial Currents, 2004. First published in 1997 by Harper-Collins Publishers.

Holland, Jimmie C. and Sheldon Lewis. *The Human Side of Cancer: Living with Hope, Coping with Uncertainty.* New York: Quill, 2001.

Hunter, Charles and Frances Hunter. *Healing Through Humor.* Lake Mary, FL: Creation House Press, 2003.

Kalick, Rosanne. *Cancer Etiquette: What to Say, What to Do, When Someone You Know or Love Has Cancer.* Scarsdale, NY: Lion Books, 2005.

Katz, Rebecca with Mat Edelson. *The Cancer-Fighting Kitchen: Nourishing, Big-Flavor Recipes for Cancer Treatment and Recovery.* Berkeley: Celestial Arts, 2009.

Klein, Allen. *The Courage to Laugh: Humor, Hope and Healing in the Face of Death and Dying.* New York: Jeremy P. Tarcher/Putnam, 1998.

Mayeroff, Milton. *On Caring.* New York: HarperPerennial, 1990. Reprint of Perennial Library edition, published in 1972.

Moore, Thomas. *Dark Nights of the Soul: A Guide to Finding Your Way Through Life's Ordeals.* New York: Penguin Group (Gotham), 2004.

National Institutes of Health. *What You Need to Know About™ Cancer* series. Bethesda: National Cancer Institute, 1994–2003.

————. *When Someone in Your Family Has Cancer.* Bethesda: National Cancer Institute, 1995.

Orchard, Anne. *Their Cancer—Your Journey: A Traveller's Guide for Carers, Family and Friends.* Charmouth, Bridport, UK: Rainbow Heart Publishing, 2008.

Outcalt, Todd. *The Healing Touch: Experiencing God's Love in the Midst of Our Pain.* Deerfield Beach, FL: Faith Communications, Inc., 2005.

Rose, Susannah L. and Richard T. Hara. *100 Questions & Answers About Caring for Family or Friends with Cancer.* Sudbury, MA: Jones and Bartlett Publishers, 2005.

Rosenbaum, Ernest H. and Isadora Rosenbaum. *Everyone's Guide to Cancer Supportive Care: A Comprehensive Handbook for Patients and Their Families.* Kansas City: Andrews McMeel Publishing, 2005.

Sheehy, Gail. *Passages In Caregiving: Turning Chaos into Confidence.* New York: William Morrow (HarperCollins), 2010.

Smith, Harold Ivan. *Grieving the Death of a Friend.* Minneapolis: Augsburg Fortress, 1996.

Zadra, Dan, compiler. *Because You Care: Celebrating Nurses, Caregivers and Other Everyday Heroes.* Lynnwood, WA: Compendium, Inc., 2005.

Zona, Guy A. *The Soul Would Have No Rainbow If the Eyes Had No Tears, and Other Native American Proverbs.* New York: Simon and Schuster, 1994.

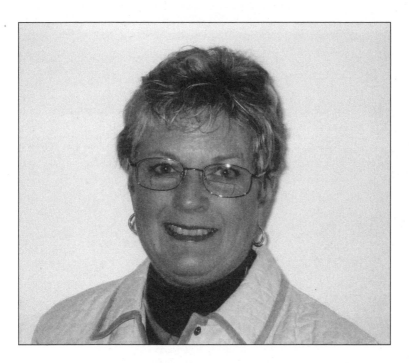

ABOUT THE AUTHOR
BONNIE E. DRAEGER, MS, MDIV

Bonnie Draeger is president and executive director of In Marjolein's Memory, Inc. (d/b/a/ Friends & Cancer) and helped cofound this public charity in 2003. She is also this book's leading contributor. Draeger counsels and supports people with cancer, leads workshops educating patients' friends and colleagues, and has served as project coordinator for *When Cancer Strikes a Friend*. She is a featured speaker on cancer survivorship, friendship and cancer, and communication during cancer.

Her work is rooted in the belief that everyone's cancer experience should be as positive and burden free as possible. As an educator and ordained United Methodist clergywoman, Rev. Draeger's life and work are dedicated to realizing this vision through the education and empowerment of friends. She cofounded Friends & Cancer in direct response to the critically important roles that friends played in her own cancer recovery.

Her first career as a music educator spanned nearly thirty years. For her work impacting the lives and education of over ten thousand children and adults, Draeger was named a 1990 "Extra-Ordinary Woman" in the State of Indiana. She has written cover articles for *Parents' Press* and *Christians in Education* and contributed to the textbook *Music: A Way of Life for the Young Child* (Charles Merrill, 1987). She has also written and published numerous articles and musical compositions.

Rev. Draeger and her husband, Wayne, live on Cape Cod, where she enjoys writing, painting, ministry, and spending time with her four young granddaughters.

To learn more about Friends & Cancer or to contact the author, please visit www.friendsandcancer.org.

ADDITIONAL CONTRIBUTORS

RACHEL ABRAM, MA, MPhil, was a freelance developmental editor, specializing in nonfiction. Based in New York City, Rachel worked with writers in a wide range of subject areas including literary and art history, biography, medicine, finance, and career development. The late Ms. Abram served as the developmental editor for *When Cancer Strikes a Friend*. She also cofounded Auburn Seminary's international youth peace initiative, Face to Face: Faith to Faith.

ELAINE M. AMERSON, EdD, is a national leadership development consultant whose involvements include the Chicago Public Schools, Urban Ministries National Consultation, and The Connectional Table of the United Methodist Church. She serves on the staff of Garrett-Evangelical Theological Seminary, Evanston, Illinois.

GENA ASHER, MIS (Master of Information Science), is creator and Webmaster of BreastCancerFYI.org. She teaches at the Indiana University School of Journalism, where she is the Web editor. Her writing and Web development have won several awards, including the Woman's Press Club of Indiana's highest honors.

STEVEN D. AVERILL, MDiv, FT, is a bereavement counselor at Hospice of the Valley (Phoenix, Arizona). He is the author of *Grief and the Healing Process: Understanding Our Losses.*

DAVID BECHHOFER and **JESSICA BECHHOFER** are a Massachusetts father-daughter cancer advocacy team. Jessica, now a college student, lost her mother to cancer at age three and a half and began walking for cancer awareness at age five. David Bechhofer founded the Susan G. Komen 3-Day Youth Corps and the Avon Walk for Breast Cancer Youth Crew, both national programs for ten- to sixteen-year-old young people.

AMY BLUMENFELD, MS, is a childhood-cancer survivor and a journalist whose articles have been published in *The New York Times, O-The Oprah Magazine, Fitness, People, Self, Marie Claire,* and other magazines. Ms. Blumenfeld has appeared on MSNBC, CBS News, and Fox News in connection with her writings and topics relating to survivorship issues. She is a former staff writer and editor at *George* magazine and *American Health* magazine.

DAN COSTIN, MD, is an oncologist, hematologist, and internist in White Plains, New York. He is the medical director of the Westchester Institute for Treatment of Cancer and Blood Disorders, where he is known for his empathic approach to the treatment of cancer. Dr. Costin is chief emeritus of the Division of Hematology and Oncology at White Plains Hospital Center. He is also comedical director of the White Plains Hospital Cancer Program.

DAVE COVERLY is the award-winning creator of the syndicated cartoon series *Speed Bump,* appearing in over 250 newspapers internationally. His cartoons have been published in *The New Yorker* and *Parade Magazine*. In 2009 he was named Outstanding Cartoonist of the Year by the National Cartoonist Society.

CAROL DECKER, PhD, MSEd, MSW, is an assistant research scientist at the Indiana University School of Nursing. Her area of expertise is research on coping, social support, and communication in families facing cancer. She is also a coauthor of the textbook, *Developing Helping Skills: A Step-by-step Approach.*

JOSEPH DISA, MD, is a plastic surgeon at Memorial Sloan-Kettering Cancer Center, New York City, who specializes in reconstruction following tumor surgery. Dr. Disa is coauthor of *100 Questions and Answers About Breast Surgery* and many professional articles.

DANIELLE FERRER, RN, is a registered nurse at Memorial Sloan-Kettering Cancer Center, New York City.

MICHAEL FINKELSTEIN, MD, is former senior vice president for medical affairs and chief of the Department of Medicine at Northern Westchester Hospital in Mount Kisco, New York. He studied integrative medicine under Dr. Andrew Weill and is the founder and director of SunRaven, a holistic health center in Bedford, New York.

ILANA FLEISHMAN, a breast cancer survivor, holds a masters degree in library and information studies, and has worked as a reference librarian in Canada.

PAMELA FOELSCH, PhD, is clinical assistant professor of psychology in psychiatry at Weill Medical College of Cornell University. Dr. Foelsch is widely published and is a featured speaker in the field of personality disorders. Her contribution draws upon her own family's cancer experiences as well as her counseling of adolescents and adults.

MELISSA GILL, MD, is a practicing dermatopathologist and medical director of SkinMedical Research and Diagnostics in Dobbs Ferry, New York. She devotes much of her time to collaborative research in dermatology and dermatopathology, and she is a recognized international specialist in the field of reflectance confocal microscopy. Dr. Gill has co-edited a textbook as well as coauthored many original articles and book chapters.

WILLIAM GRIFFITH, MDiv, DMin, is a retired chaplain of Hospice of South Central Indiana (Columbus, IN). Rev. Griffith counsels the terminally ill. He is the author of three books, *More Than a Parting Prayer: Lessons in Caregiving for the Dying, Confronting Death,* and *Tears in a Bottle: Learning How to Grieve Well.*

ALEXANDRA HEERDT, MD, is a leading breast surgeon at Memorial Sloan-Kettering Cancer Center. Dr. Heerdt appears frequently on *New York Magazine's* list of the top 100 doctors in New York City. In 2009 she received an American Cancer Society national award in recognition of her tireless commitment to the saving of lives.

DAVID JENKINS, MDiv, DMin, served in the Chaplaincy and Pastoral Education Department at M.D. Anderson Cancer Center, Houston, from 1993–2009. An ordained minister, Rev. Jenkins worked closely with cancer patients and their families until his recent retirement.

ROSANNE KALICK, MA, MLS, was professor of library science at Westchester Community College in New York, earning the State University Chancellor's Award for Excellence in Librarianship. The late Ms. Kalick authored *Cancer Etiquette: What to Say, What to Do, When Someone You Know or Love Has Cancer.*

ROSALIND KLEBAN, BS, MSW, is senior clinical supervisor at the Evelyn Lauder Breast Center, Memorial Sloan-Kettering Cancer Center. Ms. Kleban has been honored by the Susan G. Komen Foundation (Professor of Survivorship, 2004) and by the Association of Oncology Social Workers, which named her Social Worker of the Year in 2005.

KRISTIN KWAK, MS, RD, LDN, is a registered dietitian-nutrition therapist, currently in private practice in Bucks County, Pennsylvania. Ms. Kwak's specialty is integrated health and wellness.

HENRY LEE, MD, PhD, a radiation oncologist, is associate director for radiation oncology at the Dickstein Cancer Center in White Plains, New York. He is affiliated with the Westchester Institute for Treatment of Cancer and Blood Disorders in White Plains.

JULIE MEEK, DNS, RN, CNS, is clinical associate professor, Indiana University School of Nursing. She is a recent cancer survivor.

JULIE MONROE, MD, is chief of the Department of Hematology and Oncology, White Plains Hospital Center (White Plains, New York). Dr. Monroe trained at New York Presbyterian Hospital and Memorial Sloan-Kettering Cancer Center, has received awards for her academic excellence and her cancer research, and is well known for her dedication to outstanding patient care and support.

JEFFREY MUMPER, MS, is clinical physicist for the Indiana University Health Cancer Radiation Centers (Bloomington, Indiana), where he creates the computer models—"virtual patients"—of people preparing to undergo radiation therapy.

MARY C. MURPHREE, PhD, was a regional administrator in the U.S. Department of Labor for two decades, overseeing the interests of six million working women in New York, New Jersey, Puerto Rico, and the U.S. Virgin Islands. An ovarian cancer survivor, Ms. Murphree is currently a senior advisor at the Center for Women and Work at Rutgers University.

SIGRID OLSEN is a cancer survivor and nationally known artist and textile designer. Ms. Olsen holds an artist's diploma and honorary doctorate from Monseratt College. In addition to her work as an artist, she leads inspirational retreats in the United States, Europe, and Mexico.

MICHELLE Y. PEARLMAN, PhD, is a clinical psychologist in private practice in Rockland County, New York, and Northern New Jersey. She is an adjunct faculty member at the Department of Child and Adolescent Psychiatry at the NYU School of Medicine. Dr. Pearlman specializes in helping children and their families coping with grief, trauma, anxiety, and stressful life events.

SUSAN JI-ON POSTAL, MA, is an ordained Zen Buddhist priest and currently serves as teacher-in-residence at the Empty Hand Zen Center in New Rochelle, New York.

BENJAMIN A. RANCK, MD, was the medical director of Hospice of South Central Indiana (Columbus, Indiana) until 2009. A specialist in family medicine, Dr. Ranck began his hospice work in 1980 and continued this work after retiring from forty-five years of family practice.

HEATHER RICHARDSON, MD, specializes in the surgical care of breast disease in Atlanta, Georgia. She has special interest in innovative surgical techniques and genetic and environmental risk factors that can contribute to the formation of cancer.

JANICE ROSS, MSN, MA, RN, OCN®, CBCN®, has managed the Olcott Center for Cancer Education (Bloomington, Indiana) for many years. As an oncology nurse, cancer educator, and cancer survivor, Ms. Ross counsels newly diagnosed cancer patients, their families and friends. She also leads community cancer-awareness and education events.

KEVIN RUSH, MHA, RT (R)(T), is administrative director of the Indiana University Health Cancer Radiation Centers (Bloomington, Indiana). There he oversees the daily operations of the radiation oncology department.

ANJALI SAQI, MD, MBA, is an associate professor in the Department of Pathology and Cell Biology and Director of Cytopathology at Columbia University Medical Center, New York Presbyterian Hospital in New York City. She practices general surgical pathology and cytopathology and is actively involved in research and teaching, having coauthored over thirty-five peer-reviewed articles.

CATHERINE SHERWOOD-LAUGHLIN, HSD (Doctorate of Health and Safety), **MPH, MA**, is clinical associate professor in the Department of Applied Health Science, Indiana University. Dr. Sherwood's course on cancer is one of the most sought-after health science undergraduate classes, and she is widely published in the field of health sciences.

GLORIA STEADMAN-SANNERMARK, RN, MDiv, is a nurse and an ordained clergywoman. She has been a hospice chaplain and currently works with older adults in the Sun Cities of Arizona.

MARGARET (PEG) STICE, BA, is Internship Coordinator, Nonprofit Leadership Alliance, at the School of Public and Environmental Affairs, Indiana University (Bloomington). She has spent over forty years in nonprofit management, currently is chairperson of the board of directors of Friends & Cancer, and was a founding member of the organization.

MARTHA (MARTY) TOUSLEY, CNS-BC, FT, DCC, is a bereavement counselor with Hospice of the Valley, Phoenix, Arizona. She is also a registered nurse, an advanced nurse practitioner, and a mental health consultant. She is the author of *Finding Your Way Through Grief: A Guide for the First Year*.

CAROL RICHMOND TSANG, PhD, is a former assistant professor of history at the University of Illinois at Chicago and a cancer survivor. Retired from teaching, Ms. Tsang assists with not-for-profit projects, and has served on the staff of Friends & Cancer®.

INDEX

A

accepting help, 27, 106

accommodations. *See* housing assistance

adolescents, 119, 121. *See also* teens

advocacy, 68, 126, 186–188, 189, 190, 215

    activism, 68, 189, 190

health care advocate, 126, 186–187

    insurance advocate, 126

    patient advocate, 215

    ways to advocate, 186–188

alternative approaches. *See* complementary-integrative

American Cancer Society, 109, 195

American Society of Clinical Oncology, 195

anxiety, 17, 52, 110

appetite, 80, 146

art, 54–56, 112, 181, 187

attitude, 9–10, 16, 18, 22, 29–30, 119, 124, 183. *See also* emotions

    denial, 16, 22, 183

    doubt, 16, 22, 183

    optimism, 29–30

    privacy, 9–10, 119, 124

    sarcasm, 18

B

beauty during cancer, 53, 54–56

benign, 130, 208

bereavement. *See* grief

biopsies, 130–131

bladder cancer, 199